YOUR BEST BODY AFTER 45

THE ADVANCED STRENGTH TRAINING GUIDE FOR BUILDING MUSCLE AND MAXIMIZING FITNESS AT 45 AND BEYOND

BRYANT WILLIS

CONTENTS

Before we get acquainted , I'd like to tell you about a concise book I made to complement what you're about to read. The cornerstone of supreme fitness is a healthy diet. That is why I have devised a meal plan to help you lose fat and sustain a happy body.

However , I thought that pushing a sale after you just bought one of my books would be unfair and a little greedy. So, instead, I've decided to give you this one for free! Here is a little sneak preview of what value you will be getting out of this free book:

- An entire day of delicious meals laid out for you, designed specifically to help you lose fat
- Alternative meals to mix things up so you will never get bored
- Vital information on what foods to eat and ones to stay away from so you can become an expert on weight loss

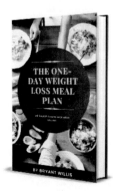

As I said, it's free, so you might as well take a look inside. It's a verystraightforward process. All you have to do is click the link below then it will take you to a page where you can type in your email, and I can send it straight to you. Here's the link...
bryantjwillis.com
I hope you love it!

If you are reading a printed version of the book , I ask you to type in bryantwillis.com into your browser and you will be directed to the same place.

Enjoy!

INTRODUCTION

"Almost everything we have been taught about aging is wrong. We now know that a very fit body of 70 can be the same as a moderately fit body of 30."

— BY DR. WALTER BORTZ, MD

Warm Up

A lot of the older people I talk to are often caught up with their age. They discover a passion for strength training, want to get their bodies into great shape, and appreciate the health benefits of being physically fit, especially after 45. Often as humans, we have enough awareness to know what is good for us and how to achieve it, yet we still fall into the traps of self-doubt. These mental blocks can manifest in many forms, and the thought of an aging body is no exception.

We see our age as the factor that decides how well our bodies can perform. In reality, one's age is simply a mental barrier. A 20-pound dumbbell doesn't care whether you are 20 years old or 75 years old; it's going to give everyone an equal amount of resistance. It's up to you, the person who is training, to figure out how well you can perform and then work out a way to get the results that transcend into a sustainable lifestyle. The only mistake you can make is getting into a program that is not in line with your fitness goals or tailored to meet your requirements.

I'm not saying your age is not relevant. It's certainly relevant, it dictates the kind of training you do and how you do it, but you mustn't let it hold you back. There is undoubtedly no problem with exercise under any age. You only need to watch how you train and how your body responds to the stimulus.

Why Age Isn't A Problem

You might have heard of Japan as one of the world's leading economies, one of the best tourist locations, or perhaps as a country that produces some of the most expensive fruit on the planet. However, you might not have heard that Japan is also home to the world's oldest population. Over a third of the Japanese population is over the age of 65.

The seniors living in Japan are among the healthiest people globally, even outside of their age group. They can live such long lives because they have an incredibly balanced and nutritious diet and maintain a highly active lifestyle.

However, healthy people are found all over the world in the senior age group. Suppose we consider the example of Jack Lalanne, who recently passed away in 2011, aged 96. If you don't know the story of Jack Lalanne, he was an American fitness and nutrition guru. You may be surprised to know that many of the feats he was well known for were performed after 40. In fact, he was setting world records well into his late 60s and even 70s.

One of the most incredible feats of strength was in 1984 when he managed to tow 70 boats loaded with 70 passengers for over a mile. This record was set at age 70! To add to this, he was handcuffed and shackled and was fighting strong winds and currents.

This is not the only record that Lalanne set. He has a long list of physical milestones that he achieved well after the age of 40. This shows that you can do anything if you have the correct preparation and planning.

Baby Steps

Everyone is in a different physical condition by the time they reach 50. Some people have had a relatively active life, while others have had a more sedentary lifestyle. Whatever scenario you find yourself in, you need a fitness program tailored to that situation. If you have some experience with strength training and are familiar with weights, using gym equipment, and calisthenics, then this is the book for you. We will look past the basics and dive deep into the art of exercise so you can push through the wall you are hitting in muscle growth and take your training to the next level.

If you are a beginner or have grown out of touch with the world of fitness, I highly suggest you read my previous book in the series, "The Seven Keys To Strength Training For Men Over 50". This book serves as an introduction to the latest information on strength training. It's the perfect way to get familiarized with basic movements, exercise mechanics, rest and recovery, and nutrition. You will learn the fundamental aspects of what it takes to build muscle and lose excess fat. After reading, you will be fully equipped and ready to move onto the second installment - Your Best Body After 45.

Making The Change

The best time to embark on a journey to a healthier version of yourself is today. Unfortunately, (as I am sure you know) it becomes harder to increase our muscle mass as the year's pass. Still, instead of letting that dictate our lives, you should find closure and satisfaction in knowing that to achieve your goals, you work harder than any 20-year-old.

It's going to take persistence if you want to prevent that arthritis from flaring up, if you're going to see progress like you used to, and if you wish to chisel your abdominals into the ideal shape.

Apart from the physical difficulties that people face in their 50's and 60's, the mental struggles are just as challenging, if not more so. Your self-worth, self-image, and even ability to look at life in a positive light can start to deteriorate if we let it. What's worse is people often exaggerate the severity of their physical condition in their minds. Just because you experience pain in your wrists from arthritis doesn't mean you have to stop doing push-ups. Or another one I hear a lot about is people who have diabetes thinking they can't eat what they want to. These are only some of the problems I try to help my clients work through.

In most cases, understanding your diet and training in the gym or at home has helped people naturally cure the problems they faced and decreased their reliance on medications and treatments. You drastically improve joint and bone health and even stabilize insulin sensitivity through a proper diet and a thorough training regimen.

This book is designed specifically to meet the requirements of people of your age. I understand what you need, and I know how to help best you get maximum results.

The Journey

It's not going to be easy; it never is. Whether you are 18 or 80, physical training is never a simple job. How can it be when the only way to build muscle requires you to create micro-tears in your muscles so they grow back stronger. When you set a personal best on the bench press, its weight you have never lifted before, it takes a level of effort that you have never exerted before! So, of course, it's going to be challenging.

But is it worth it?

In my personal experience, and in the experience of the countless number of people that I have trained with, the simple answer is YES, one hundred times out of one hundred. Even though it's tough when you are in the trenches, it's always worth it when you come out the other side victorious.

As with everything else in life, the journey of body transformation is fueled by consistency and discipline. Especially after that initial 12 to 16 weeks of training, when you feel like your muscle growth has started to plateau, you begin to lose motivation. At this point, you need to remember that Setbacks are part of the process; you only truly fail when you choose not to get up again. This is the time to pick yourself up and stay zeroed in, pushing past that barrier using all the dedication you can muster. If you can accomplish this, then the feeling of success will positively affect your life in a big way.

You will love how people start seeing you differently, and the positive energy will radiate to every part of your life outside the gym. There's a beautiful life waiting for you down this path. All you have to do is listen to my advice down to the finest detail.

A Bit About Me

From as far back as I can remember, I have loved physical sports and activities. I always enjoyed playing team sports as a kid, such as soccer. As I got older, I introduced myself to strength training naturally as I grew more and more involved in martial arts. My focus shifted from team sports to working out in the gym. As time passed, I realized my passions lay in strength training and my goal of becoming an international mixed martial artist. I then used the knowledge I gained to help others as a personal trainer and coach. Over the years, I have worked with various individuals, ranging from total beginners to top-tier athletes.

However, my focus has leaned towards training people in their mid-life and above. I see so many in this age group continuing down the path of unhealthy life choices because society sidelines them simply because of their age. I believe there is no right age to change your body and improve your health, there is only the right time, and that time is right now.

So, let me first congratulate you on taking another big step to a better life; let's get started.

Me As Your Trainer

Physical training varies greatly depending on your goals and, more importantly, where you are starting from. Training someone who is 50 years old is very different from training a 22-year-old. That is undeniable, but no need to worry. I have made it my specialty to train people of your age group, so you can sit comfortably knowing that everything I teach is within your best interests.

My ideologies are rooted in the latest science, and this book translates them acutely. More than just telling you what to do and how to do it, I'm all about educating my athletes and telling them why they are doing what they are doing. Not only does this make it a lot more interesting for the reader/trainee, but it also helps you understand the laws of exercise so you can make decisions about your training confidently.

Throughout this book, we will look at the best workout strategies designed for maximum muscle growth, an in-depth analysis of different gym equipment, and how to incorporate it into your life, regardless of injuries and diseases.

If you wish to get in shape for summer, then go to the gym. If you desire to be healthy for the rest of your life, then understand this book and internalize the core concepts so that a healthy body becomes an extension of yourself rather than a constant struggle.

To summarise, I want to convey the more advanced information that will resonate specifically with your strength training goals. Whether you choose to use bodyweight or free weights at home or in the gym, there is something for everyone.

To get the most value from this book, I highly suggest you make notes of key points and go over things that you will be using multiple times. If you have something in particular that you want to focus on, and you want to skip ahead, then be my guest. Although let me make it known that going through the whole book will bring you around to some new opportunities and open your mind up to some practices you may not have considered.

There is a lot to go through, so let's get the ball rolling. I'll see you in the first chapter...

TRAINING SMART IN YOUR LATER 40'S AND BEYOND:
INJURIES AND ILLNESSES NEED NOT DRAG YOU DOWN

THE PIT

What's a common theme between a UFC main event, a formula one race, and a commercial flight?

They all have to go through a systems check. Fighters get a medical examination, weigh-in, and get their hand wraps examined right before the bout. Formula one cars are checked just before the race, tires are heated up, and the engine is tested for any faults. Commercial flights have a similar process for both the plane and the pilots. Everyone and everything is critically evaluated before an aircraft is allowed to leave the ground.

All three of these examples require absolute perfection to perform their goal without anything going wrong. I want you to take the same approach when it comes to your strength training.

Whether you've been continuously in the gym for the past few years or you're returning to the weight room after some time on the sidelines. Before you get started, you need to evaluate your health. Especially now in your later years, you need to have a clear understanding of the strengths and weaknesses of your body. While strength training is the goal, we also want to achieve overall fitness and improve the general condition of your body. If physical fitness and wellness are the destinations, then strength training is the path.

DIAGNOSTICS

With a lot of the clients that I have worked with, I have found that not understanding the physical condition of your body before starting a fitness regimen has resulted in more injuries and problems. Many people who train without a trainer's guidance or simply a friend to watch them will continuously exercise with poor form for years. Without anyone telling you something is wrong, you will develop a habit, and after years of adopting that habit, it becomes challenging to shake it off.

This lack of understanding leads to excessive stress on the joints and tendons. For instance, I often see people with the wrong hand placement on the bar when doing a bench press. Over a few years, they can develop chronic wrist problems and tennis elbow issues. Naturally, they conclude that it is a bone condition and treat it with anti-inflammatory drugs. Even doctors may treat it, considering it a bone or joint problem, never realizing that it's due to poor form when working out. Especially when you are lifting several hundred pounds or the equivalent to your body weight, it places a tremendous amount of stress on these joints and the associated tendons and ligaments.

Whether you have been regularly lifting for the past 20 years or getting back into the gym after five years off, we need to know exactly where you stand in physical fitness. It will help us decide how you can make the most gains possible and create a workout that is guaranteed to help you improve your health.

Ideally, you should consult with a doctor and discuss your plans about moving forward with a strength training protocol. Also, it would be best if you shared the workout with a reliable and trusted trainer. Talk to your trainer about any medical conditions you have had or are still battling today. Whether that is a sprained ankle that acts up from time to time or an open-heart surgery you had a couple of years ago, realize that this is critical information moving forward.

It's unlikely that you will find the right trainer or doctor the first time around, but don't give up. Keep looking around, researching, and talking to people you think might be a good fit for you. That could even be a trusted friend, one that is knowledgeable in the world of fitness.

Medical reports are relatively straightforward to deal with; they provide an unbiased finding of what is happening in your body. Whether that is a detailed blood sugar report or an X-ray of a joint, with this information on hand, you can move towards developing training routines that work around these problems and help improve them.

I 100% advise that you check in with a doctor, but I also understand that many people can't afford a trainer, so don't worry, you don't have to get one. Although I believe an excellent trainer goes a long way, it's important to note that many of the so-called "experts" out there are more interested in how big your wallet is rather than how big your gains are. It's unfortunate, but it's the truth these days. So, if you want to skip the part where you find a good trainer, it's fine with me as long as you follow this book and pay attention to your body.

In terms of getting your form correct and making sure you are doing things properly; you can simply get a friend to watch you. For those who prefer to work out alone, record yourself performing exercises and then relay the tape to see if it looks acceptable. It's often difficult to evaluate your form when you are focused on the movement, but you can identify areas that need improvement by watching yourself do it. An even better approach is sharing the video of you exercising with more experienced lifters who can give you their expert feedback.

Getting expert advice doesn't have to be costly. You can share your workout videos in our Facebook group "Strength And Fitness For The Aged Warriors" and get feedback from members who are seasoned trainers and expert lifters. It's is a place where many of my clients and colleagues come together to share our passion for strength training, and it's an environment that provides support to all kinds of lifters. I will personally provide you with help on everything from your workout to your diet. Check it out by typing in the name of our group on Facebook and see for yourself.

WELCOME TO THE "NEW SCHOOL"

Remember when "no pain, no gain" was the motto of every bodybuilder, strength athlete, and even the receptionist at your local gym. Well, times haven't changed, they were wrong then, and they are still wrong today.

That is probably the worst piece of advice you could give anyone. Think about it. Is a torn Achilles good progress? Is a ripped bicep good for your arms? Would you classify a damaged lower back due to poor deadlift posture as good 'gains'?

These are the kind of gains that are going to put you in a hospital bed for six months and most probably spell the end of your strength training career. The only thing you will be gaining is an enormous medical bill and more time to think about how wrong your decision was to lift using the power of your ego.

Starting today, let's reinterpret the "no pain no gain" motto in a new light and put a positive spin on it.

Discipline is the real pain when it comes to getting in top physical condition, losing fat, packing on muscle, getting to the gym day in and day out, and eating right.

The only pain you need to be concerned about is the pain of getting up in the early morning to get your cardio in. The pain of not eating what's readily available. The pain of putting your meals together beforehand and sticking to your diet. The pain of spending the time necessary to correct any incorrect movements you might have become accustomed to over the years.

Okay, so it might sound like I'm ranting, but if you wish to grow into a better version of yourself, one that people admire, you must exercise discipline, and it needs to come from you because I do not have the power to change that. My soul purpose with this book is to help you reduce the physical pains one experiences. Arthritis, osteoporosis, diabetes, blood pressure, osteoarthritis, and the list goes on.

Yes! It's possible. We can solve all these issues, and many others like them, through strength training and proper nutrition. Remember, most of these problems either arise or are exaggerated due to an imbalance in the body; by bringing you back to equilibrium, we can offset the discomfort these conditions create.

AGE AND COMMON PROBLEMS

You might have already noticed that as we age the body starts to weaken. Even if you have led a relatively healthy lifestyle, it becomes more challenging to maintain muscle mass and recovery takes longer. Most of your friends around the 50-year mark are all going to be complaining about some physical problem or the other.

In my experience, some of the most common problems I have seen with clients include:

- Tennis elbow
- Osteoarthritis
- Osteoporosis
- Hearing loss
- Cardiovascular diseases
- Blood pressure
- Diabetes
- Arthritis

While these are naturally occurring problems, there are also many problems that people have to face as a result of an accident, or an extreme medical condition. Limited mobility, poor vision, reduced motor control, and other similar issues are also common.

Most, if not all, of these problems, are directly related to age. There is simply a higher chance of them happening, and a greater acuteness with which they happen as we age. However, while we can't eliminate them entirely, there are things we can do to minimize their impact and keep them under control without medications and treatments.

Their Connection To Training

Whether it is a disease you are having trouble with or a problem with your joint or muscle, the situation's impact on your training will vary. Most of these problems and other similar issues that men face as they approach their fifties and beyond are going to impact the health of your joints, nerves, bones, and cardiovascular system. Thorough strength training relies on these elements to train the body to develop muscle mass, reduce fat and develop higher overall strength.

If left untreated, the impact of these problems can be shown in your reaction times, flexibility, balance, base strength levels, and endurance. Even though I believe exercise is a necessary treatment, it cannot be denied that some conditions inhibit your ability to work out and limits the rate of progress you can expect to make.

Though this doesn't mean you won't or can't make progress at all.

THE DEVIL'S IN THE DETAIL

If you have a bad shoulder, you might be able to do cardio for hours, but you will have trouble lifting anything overhead. The solution is to work around the problem, strengthen the shoulder, activate the smaller surrounding muscles that support your shoulder, and use an exercise to directly train that muscle group without placing too much stress on the joint. It's also essential to discover why and how that shoulder is causing you discomfort and what kind of medical intervention can improve your condition. While we don't want medicines to be the long-term solution, they play a vital role in relieving the initial pain while building structure through light training.

Our primary focus may not be to use strength training as therapy for physical problems; it is to develop strength, but a beneficial side effect is that you will see a lot of improvement in these issues.

For instance, if you face trouble with diabetes, strength training and proper nutrition can go a long way in leveling out your blood sugar levels. Quite obviously, if you can control the kind of food you eat, you have a lot more control over how much sugar is in your blood-stream. Secondly, as you train and use more energy, you can more effectively channel the excess sugar in your body by doing intensive exercise. Your body uses energy by burning glucose in the form of pyruvate. However, it's not an easy task, it does take continuous effort, but it's a lot of fun and much more rewarding than having to inject yourself every time you sit down to eat.

Let me emphasize that you need to get a good medical checkup before you start training. I have had clients in the past who had been facing gastrointestinal issues for years with no idea why it's happening, and they never sought any medical attention because they lacked consideration of the problem. Before they began training, they consulted with a doctor and found out they were lactose intolerant. They had been eating dairy-based diets all along and simply changing that one area of their diet helped them alleviate years of further discomfort.

So, if you have any physical or mental problems, consider strength training as a natural remedy. While it may not entirely solve the issue, it is a very potent addition to any medicines or treatments you may be having.

ADDITIONAL BENEFITS

A healthy body is a result of not only being physically fit but also mentally nourished and balanced. Sports play a massive role, especially in strength training where you are competing against yourself. You are entirely reliant on yourself, and the enemy is also none other than the man or woman standing in the mirror.

It's important to understand that the path to building a more robust and healthier physique does not come by converging on a single area. If you struggle with over-head press, the problem isn't necessarily limited to your shoulders; your lower back and legs may also have a part to play.

With a strength training program that helps you develop your entire body, you can start making rapid gains. Especially if you have been training for a while but have developed injuries due to improper technique or incorrect training, managing those problems is vital.

The benefits of strength training are ubiquitous. The results are fantastic, especially when you complement a training routine with the proper nutrition and supplements.

I've come across several people over the years who had problems that, on the surface, seemed like they had nothing to do with strength training, or at least were issues that didn't seem fixable by training. One of the essential things that deteriorate with age is the quality and quantity of sleep. Surprisingly, I've had clients and friends come back to me stating their sleep has improved tremendously. Their improved quality of sleep is helping them wake up refreshed, more relaxed, and in a much more positive state of mind. People have seen improvements in their cardiovascular health through strength training, they have fought off depression and anxiety, and many have developed more discipline in their lives.

This is because strength training is such as demanding sport. The effects it has on athletes often benefit them in many areas of life. Simply by getting yourself onto the path of strength training, you are getting involved in a life improvement project. You are working on everything, including physical conditioning, exercise, mental toughness, nutrition, and, most importantly, my favorite word (as I'm sure you've guessed by now), discipline.

Getting Results

there has to be a reason why you chose to invest in this book, and it's either because you can't get the results you're looking for or the program you are in isn't sustainable. People often get on a program that is either too advanced for them or too basic. They eventually can't keep up with the requirements or lose motivation because they aren't getting the desired results, making them fall off track for months. Be honest with me. Has this happened to you at some point? A good program is sufficiently challenging, produces results, and is easy to follow given your resources and circumstances.

Let's look at a few things you can implement immediately to get the results you are looking for more efficiently.

1. Warm-Up/Cool-Down

While you must do the actual weightlifting with proper form and technique, it's also vital that you give your body the room to properly warm-up and cool-down before and after a workout. Especially with the stress you are subjugating your body to, it's vital that your entire body is warmed up, has good blood flow into each muscle, and is ready to exert itself. A good warm-up can be done by performing simple dynamic exercises like high kicks and jumping jacks to get the blood pumping.

After the workout, foam rolling, cold showers, and stretching are essential in helping the muscles cool down and promote recovery. Lastly, for your sake, do not perform any static stretches before a workout. I see this too often, and it is a terrible practice. Recent studies have shown that static stretches right before exercise can tire out the muscles, which can be detrimental to your performance. I also believe it increases your chance of injury. So please do me a favor by saving the static stretches for after.

2. Training Weak Spots

If you are having problems with certain areas, maybe an achy joint or perhaps a muscle that has not yet recovered, you need to devise ways to work around that weakness or consider not training it at all for some time. In most cases, it can be helpful to stretch the affected area regularly and perform low-intensity exercises to build up strength.

3. Supplements

You may consider protein as the be-all and end-all, as most trainees do. However, I suggest you consider investing in others such as multivitamins, probiotics, and especially fish oil. Research has proven fish oil to be highly effective for both fat loss and joint health. Moreover, the high omega-three fatty acid content has also been very beneficial for cardiovascular health. Consult with your doctor or a pharmacist before getting any supplements, then consider making these a part of your regular diet.

These are just a few of the things you could be doing differently. If you keep reading, we will explore the many avenues you can take to improve your physique. For now, let's discuss specific things you can do to train effectively and safely with various medical conditions.

WEIGHT TRAINING WITH CARDIOVASCULAR PROBLEMS

Heart disease was relatively rare just a few decades ago, but today even people as young as 20 are diagnosed with cardiovascular problems. This rise in cases is primarily due to poor nutrition and excess fat, sugar, and fast-food consumption. Combined with a sedentary lifestyle, it results in a recipe for disaster. While some cardiovascular diseases and conditions are very crippling in the sense that the patient is physically limited to what they can do, other conditions like angina can significantly be improved through physical activity.

While walking and swimming are often recommended for people with heart conditions, strength training can be a powerful game-changer if you know how to do it right.

However, there are a few exceptions.

There are certain heart conditions in which it is not advisable to participate in strength training or weightlifting. If you suffer from severe pulmonary congestion, uncontrolled blood pressure, or are at risk of congestive heart failure, you should stay away from weight training for the time being.

Even if you don't have these specific problems but do have some form of cardiovascular problem, it's highly recommended that you keep your training MODER-ATE. If you have been training in the recent past, then ideally, you should start with a weight that is lighter than what you're used to and then work your way up. Especially when you are just beginning, you want to keep the load light and measure how your body reacts to the weight. Your mind may be telling you to add more, but don't be tempted. You wouldn't eat a steak by shoving the whole thing in your mouth; you take it one bite at a time and enjoy it.

Also, keep in mind that just because you are hitting the weight room doesn't mean you shouldn't spend time on the treadmill or in the pool. Getting enough cardio is extremely important and beneficial for those with cardiovascular problems. Make sure you can strike a healthy balance between both forms of exercise.

Also, when training with weights, be sure not to hold your breath. When strength training, we are often tempted to do this when pushing or pulling a heavy load.

If you enjoy a pre-workout meal, as some people do, try to keep it light and easy to digest. You don't want to have all your blood in your gut; it should be readily available for muscles and the heart. Lastly, staying hydrated during the workout is essential, even more so if you are already in a hot and humid environment.

TRAINING WITH BACK PAIN

Back pain is one of those things that everyone has experienced at some point or other in life. Whether you just woke up on the wrong side of the bed or it's a result of a heavy deadlifting session, back pain is never enjoyable.

While back pain could simply arise from stress and fatigue, lack of sleep, or even spending too many hours sitting down, it could also indicate a deep-seated problem (no pun intended). If you haven't had your back pain adequately examined by a medical expert, you certainly want to have this done before going full steam ahead with strength training.

Back pain can be an indicator of arthritis and many other bone-related problems. If this is the case, you want to find out exactly why you are having this problem to create a workout that will help reduce the pain.

For instance, long-term lifters, especially those who squat heavy weights, can have problems where the sections of the spine get fused together. On the other end of the spectrum are those who lift with bad posture and then develop excessive gaps between spine segments. In both cases, the result is pain... and a lot of it. But the treatment for these conditions is very different. Without an accurate evaluation of the problem, you can't develop a workout routine to prevent further damage.

On the contrary, there are several exercises you can do in the gym that will improve spine health and even solve muscle-related problems in your back. For example - the side plank and curl up are great for engaging the muscles needed for excellent spine stability. Again, this is another reason you should have an expert trainer and doctor to consult with to get the most out of your exercise routine and improve your health.

ACTION PLAN

Now that you better understand medical conditions and their relevance to your strength training goals let's dive into a few things you can do today to set yourself up for success in the gym.

Start In The Kitchen

Whether you want to gain weight or lose it, your diet will help you achieve that goal. Starting today, work out an estimate for how many calories you need depending on your intention. It doesn't have to be exact because if you are eating the right food, it shouldn't matter too much; however, it will give you a better understanding of what your body is consuming. Then, plan your meals to accompany your vision for weight management. I know it sounds like hard work, and it is; however, if you are serious about making improvements, this is the place to start. It doesn't mean you can't have a greasy burger or a chocolate ice cream now and then. I'm not evil. But try your best to keep this on a special occasion basis. If you struggle with ideas or feel a bit lazy, I have constructed a weight loss meal plan to get you started. After you get bored, you can use it as inspiration to create your meal plans. If you are interested, all you have to do is head to the front of the book (just before the introduction) and follow the instructions laid out for you.

Your Team

I highly suggest finding a trainer or friend you can work with and a doctor you consult with. Ideally, these will be people who have experience in fitness and exercise. These are people you will be interacting with reasonably frequently, so more than just their portfolio; You want to find people with whom you genuinely get along and enjoy spending time. Even if you are a professional athlete with years of training experience, having an expert team is always worth it.

Homework

In closing this chapter, I want to give you some actionable advice that I hope you fulfill. If you haven't recently, I kindly ask to get your medical history in order and get a complete medical evaluation if you aren't sure about your health. Most doctors and hospitals offer a full head-to-toe checkup. If you have any recurring problems, get these checked up and relay this information to your trainer or a knowledgeable friend.

Prepare

Using the information you receive after consulting with a doctor, you should know precisely what you need to achieve, how you will accomplish it.

THE BOTTOM LINE

I won't lie to you. We can't prepare for all occasions, so learning to adjust and deal with these bumps in the road will be crucial.

Even though you have your own set of challenges to deal with, there is always a way around the problem, and through effective planning, you can achieve whatever you set your mind to.

Moreover, I hope that you now think of strength training in a new light. For it's not just a means of getting a great-looking body but also a way to keep you healthy and support your way of life.

With that said, let's move on to arguably the most critical and challenging part of any athlete's life, food, and nutrition.

2

NUTRITION AND SUPPLEMENTATION
FOR LIFE-LONG STRENGTH

THE HARD TRUTH

Many people tend to confuse eating clean with eating healthy, whereas they are entirely different things. While boiled rice and grilled chicken breast are great at providing you with protein and carbs, that's pretty much all that they offer. This isn't exactly a highly nutritious meal, it is clean and will give your body what is required to grow muscle, but it isn't everything your body needs.

The thing is, young people will progress relatively well even if their diet is weak. In the earlier stages of life, your body can deal with a lot more dietary punishment (which is a good thing because most youths eat like shit, if I'm honest). If you trained hard and only ate fast food and drank soft drinks, you made gains. Nothing compared to someone with a healthy diet but still significant. Unfortunately, you cannot afford this luxury any longer; that is precisely why this chapter is crucial in a book.

As we get older, many things change, and even minor changes in diet can have an evident impact. Regardless of how hard you train; the effects of a poor diet will begin to show. Even something as simple as not getting in enough water can make a considerable difference.

Why You Can't Take Nutrition Lightly

Making strength gains relies heavily on consistently eating the right food, but it also depends on the health of your body. More than just your muscles, you need to fuel your nervous system, your organs, your bones, and taste buds. Eating bland, protein-focused food all the time gets incredibly dull, trust me. Furthermore, it can be challenging for your body to use if it isn't getting the vitamins, minerals, salts, and hydration needed.

Other than diseases, medical conditions, and lifestyle changes, the overall wear and tear on our bodies drastically alter what our bodies need and how our bodies process the fuel we provide it.

One of the most significant physical changes in our bodies as it ages is the digestive system. Your stomach,

intestines, gallbladder, liver, and several other components that play a pivotal role in the digestive process,
start to weaken. The body's overall ability to absorb
nutrients diminishes significantly. As harsh of reality as
this is, there is a way around it.

Another limiting factor in physical development and a
reason for the degradation of the body is a slower
metabolism. It's a natural consequence of aging. Just
like how hormone production reduces, our
metabolism also declines. People who used to eat eight
hearty meals every day with a couple of protein
shakes during their workout find it difficult to
stomach even half of what they used to just a
decade ago.

Similarly, ongoing health conditions you might face,
such as blood pressure, diabetes, and arthritis, also
influence what and how much you can eat. Many
people who disregard or are unaware of this reality are
often the victims of these problems like:

- uncontrollable blood pressure.
- Never-ending heart problems.
- Plateau with their training no matter how hard
  they train.

Diet plays a notable role in treating several medical conditions, and what you put on your plate could either be medicine or poison for your body.

If you don't cook for yourself, I highly advise you to give it a go. Not only will you gain more control over what you eat, but it's a fantastic form of therapy. Moreover, it's a great way to stay focused on your training; it's almost like an extension to the work you put into the gym. Simply cooking your own food will help you stay on track with your physical training. I can testify, along with many others, to how gratifying it is to sit down after a hard day at the gym to eat a meal prepared for yourself.

THE FOUNDATIONS FOR A GOOD DIET

Okay, so at this point, you are probably sick of listening to me explaining the importance of a good diet, and I hope by now you are thoroughly convinced, so let's move on to some rules you can implement in the kitchen. Unlike most other sports, the aim for strength athletes is to consume as many calories as possible in order to gain as much mass as possible. While there is a significant emphasis on protein to promote muscle growth, it's really just about getting maximum energy for your body. Moreover, unlike bodybuilding, where athletes generally have a bulking and then a cutting phase, we don't emphasize leaning out.

If you have spent the last decade or two on a pure powerlifting diet, chances are, you aren't in the best shape of your life. You can most likely move a lot of weight, but you are a burden on the weighing scale and have to overeat to keep up with your body's high demand. It's a worthy endeavor to be as strong as you can be, but not at the cost of your health.

You want to keep the gains coming, you want the strength to continue to rise, but you want to do it through a less taxing lifestyle on the body. To achieve this goal, there are a few things you can keep an eye out for. These pointers will not only help you develop a better-looking physique, but it's going to reduce the unnecessary stress on your body significantly. I will try my best to make eating less of a chore for you and turn it into an enjoyable learning experience.

Protein

Humans love meat (apart from all the vegetarians and vegans out there, of course), especially if it's in the form of a nice juicy steak, smothered in butter, served with a heavy serving of mash. Maybe you like fried chicken, perhaps you are more of a burger guy, or enjoy exotic meats like elk meat or ox meat. The good news is you may still indulge in your favorite protein source. However, when it comes to meat, the vital thing to remember is leaner is better.

If you like steaks, consider choosing a leaner cut of meat with less fat, which is cooked less calorie-intensive. The same applies to any protein you enjoy; try to get a leaner version. Some of you may not like this but consider fish and seafood. It's a potent source of protein that synthesizes much better with human muscle. There are many ways you could prepare seafood, giving you abundant amounts of variety. It eliminates the tedious actions of eating the same dry chicken day in and day out, and to save you the hassle of thinking about it, fish are all very lean sources of protein.

Processed Foods

It's ubiquitous to find people who have invested in resistance training but counteract the benefits with a 'junk food' diet. Whether that's candy, crisps, or fast food, it becomes an addiction. While it's great for the calories, it offers nothing more than that. I'm sure most people know this, and I understand most people only chase processed food for flavor and the experience, nothing else.

Sugar is often painted as the evil villain when discussing weight loss compared to the tons of other ingredients, chemicals, and artificial additives you consume through processed food. However, the gravity of the situation is a lot greater than people think. I feel bad for sugar because it gets a lot of the blame, but if we take a closer look at artificial preservatives found in possessed food, we discover a disturbing truth.

Preservatives are used to ensure a longer shelf life for processed foods, but excessive consumption can weaken heart tissue, which is especially severe for aged people. Some artificial preservatives, including nitrites, have been shown to increase the risk of colon cancer. As you can see, processed foods are not to be taken lightly.

GET THE RIGHT CALORIES

Remember when I said eating clean isn't necessarily eating healthy? Well, the same can be said for calories. Just because you are within your caloric boundaries for the day doesn't always mean you are getting the right balance. It continues to be one of the big problems with processed foods; they fill you up with empty calories.

As a rule of thumb, any food or drink that gets its calories from sugar, trans fats, oils, alcohol, or even artificial sweeteners, is a source of empty calories.

If you are unfamiliar with the term empty calories, let me elaborate. They will supply you with energy and count towards your calorie intake but have little to no value in terms of nutrition. My advice is to concentrate less on adding all those calories and focus on high-value foods.

Fiber

If you have been on a dense, mass-gaining diet at any point in your life, you will have noticed that it can be pretty difficult to process this food. It's delicious, it's nutritious, but it's a burden on your digestive system, especially when you are eating five or more of these meals a day. Some people even use laxatives in their diet so that they can make room faster.

Fiber is your best friend. As we get older, we get into a health conundrum. One on hand, your digestive system is getting weaker. On the other hand, your body needs more protein to compensate for the natural rate of muscle loss and the higher protein requirement for building muscle. This problem can be solved using my good ol' friend - fiber.

Adding fiber to your diet will help you digest food much better, and it's a natural medicine for easing stomach pains. You don't need to use any pills or over-the-counter medication to improve your digestion when simply adding a couple of bowls of salad and some fruit will do the job more effectively.

A Balanced Diet

Essentially, a balanced diet has to have four key elements. It should be:

- Easy to prepare - so you don't struggle with food prep every day and save time.
- Tasty - so that you look forward to eating and don't lose commitment.
- Effective – it meets your daily macro requirements, so you are making progress with strength training.
- Efficient – it nourishes your body and improves your overall health.

Possibly the most rewarding thing about a well-balanced diet is allowing you the space to eat for pleasure on occasion, whether you like ice cream, deep-fried fast food, or just a box of doughnuts. Excessive use is where it becomes harmful. As long as your diet is in check, it won't hurt to indulge in these pleasures now and then.

Also, getting all your nutrients from various food such as a mix of protein sources, grains, legumes, fruits, and vegetables will open you up to many meal possibilities. This diversity is going to help with taste and effectiveness for your body.

Important Diet Considerations In Your 50s

Mounting research proves that the recommended daily allowance (RDA) of protein is insufficient for older adults. It's also important to note that the RDA of protein is for the maintenance of the average individual. It doesn't consider a person who is in strength training and needs more protein to stimulate growth. Surprisingly, staying at the maintenance level will cause you to lose muscle mass due to age and the fact that you are training.

Moreover, muscle development also depends on the protein you consume and how well it is synthesized in the body. As stated earlier, one of the other reasons seafood is so great is that it synthesizes exceptionally well. If you consumed 50 grams of protein from beef and the same amount of salmon, you would get a higher percentage of those 50 grams to manifest in your body from the fish.

Out of the different protein sources, protein powders are also an excellent solution. This is due to the rate at which they get into the bloodstream.

Being a strength trainee, you want to ensure that you receive the right amount of protein and get it from the most valuable sources.

Further, you need to streamline your eating patterns and keep them consistent to make the best progress. Eating smaller, more frequent meals is far more effective than eating two or three substantial meals in a day. Here is my evidence to support this claim:

1. It will be easier to eat and digest when you have a lower quantity to process.
2. With more efficient digestion, you will be able to absorb more nutrients from the meal.
3. Eating smaller, more frequent meals will keep you energized evenly throughout the day.

To continue my point, there is a general theory that eating smaller meals more frequently can help to raise your metabolism. You might hear this in older books, but unfortunately, current science has found very little proof to suggest this is factual. Although it may be a myth, you can find closure from knowing that eating smaller meals frequently throughout the day will most likely decrease your hunger and prevent you from overeating. (This is interesting because it may have been how the myth originated).

You will be putting in a lot of effort in the gym to break down muscle, and the same can be said for the level of effort you put into fueling your body. If there are large parts of the day when your body isn't getting the proper nutrients to fuel growth, it's going to start attacking muscle to get the fuel it needs. This means not eating on time will cause your body to attack existing muscles to find energy. That's why it's common for body-builders to get up after two or three hours of sleep to get a quick meal before heading back to their bed. They are constantly providing the body with energy so it won't attack existing energy sources. This method is rather extreme, and I do not follow it myself, but reflect on this point if you plan to exercise today.

Supplements

We've all seen the commercials, read about them in the papers, and heard about them in videos, but which ones are right for you?

More importantly, which ones are even safe to use? There are many kinds of supplements and many manufacturers, making it hard to choose at times. You must select the right type from a reliable source because some manufacturers aren't dependable and show low safety standards.

You need to be aware of everything you put in your body, and fitness supplements are no exception because they can often contain very harmful ingredients. Moreover, they usually rely on substances and components that are artificially made.

Many of the more popular and widely used brands are successful because they have been in the business for quite a while, and people have successfully been using their products for decades. However, these companies are also very open about their production techniques, the various standards they adhere to, and the kinds of ingredients they use.

On the other hand, you can encounter the no-name brands with little reputation but high demand due to their low selling points. One of the main reasons they can offer the same product at a much lower price is the quality of their materials. This won't make much difference if you buy a chair with inferior wood to save some extra money. However, when you buy a supplement that can have irreparable effects on your internal organs, it's a serious red flag.

I would suggest that even if you choose a fundamental supplement such as fish oil, you go with the best quality you can afford. Rather than eating three capsules a day, you should only need one if the quality is high. Lower quality fish oils have lower omega three and omega six and instead are loaded with fillers. The higher quality brands will give you more essential oils per capsule; plus, they use better-filtered oils, which means that the actual quality of the essential oils is much higher.

Some lower-quality supplement manufacturers use ingredients that are frowned upon and even banned by many sports organizations. This warning shows how dangerous it can be to use these supplements. It might seem like a cost-effective solution today, but it can have some costly repercussions down the line that requires you to pay with your health.

Before you get any supplements, you must discuss them with your doctor or a pharmacist. Especially if you are already taking medication, you don't want to start taking a supplement that will react with your prescription drugs or worsen the situation.

Liquids

The fact that protein powders have been around for so many years and are consistently used by athletes and regular people alike stands testament to it being one of the best supplements you can invest in. As the name suggests, these are SUPPLEMENTS and should be consumed alongside a healthy diet. They are by no means a replacement for real food. Ideally, it would help if you were drinking a protein powder drink twice a day. It is especially effective as a post-workout drink before your post-workout meal.

Recent studies have shown that men in their 70s experienced a drastic increase in strength after using whey protein powders. If you are using whey protein hydrolysate (WPH), it can be highly effective. WPH has already undergone partial hydrolysis (a chemical breakdown due to a reaction with water), making it very easy for your body to digest. It is the same kind of whey protein used in baby milk powder and various medicines. Overall, whey protein supplements are easy to use, inexpensive, and can be a great way to get in some extra protein. For anyone who is wondering, whey is the liquid left after milk has strained or curdled. I know it sounds gross so try not to think about it too much.

Let me share with you a couple of my favorite protein shake recipes that I use daily.

1. Fruity Gains (My Morning Shake)

Ingredients

- 1 cup pineapple juice (or chunks)
- 1 cup strawberries

- 1 medium banana
- 1 cup ice
- 1 scoop protein powder (chocolate flavor doesn't work too well with fruits)

Process

Throw everything into a juicer and blend it all up.

I usually have this in the morning, just after my fasted cardio while making breakfast. I keep the protein low in the mornings, but you could always add another scoop to make it more potent. Secondly, if you have diabetes or generally don't like anything too sweet, you could replace the pineapple juice with orange juice or simply use water instead. If you enjoy milk, that's also a great option. Again, I like to keep it light and refreshing, so I use juice.

2. Mug Of Gains (My Post-workout)

Ingredients

- ½ cup almonds (or three tablespoons of almond butter)
- 1 medium banana
- Stevia to taste (or honey)

- 1.5 cups of water
- 2 scoops of protein powder (vanilla works great)
- ½ cup of ice

Process

Combine in a juicer and blend

As a post-workout meal, this helps me stay full until my dinner is ready, and it's loaded with everything you need right after a workout. I would stick to water rather than milk to digest faster and get the protein to the muscles as soon as possible!

ACTION PLAN

When getting your nutrition in order, the first thing on your list should be understanding how many calories you need to maintain muscle mass and how many more you need to grow. (Remember, there is a difference). You can easily do this through any free online BMI calculator. Secondly, you need to convert this information into a macro breakdown to know how much protein, carbs, and fat you need in your diet. Ideally, you should consult with a trusted trainer, but if you don't have one, don't worry; you are more than capable of doing it yourself. As a general rule of thumb, consuming 0.8 grams of protein per pound of body weight every day is acceptable. You can break this down to the number of meals you consume, and that will give you a ballpark figure of how much you should be aiming for with each meal. However, please consider the calories you are consuming because it's all for nothing if they have little nutritional value. With these things in mind, you can move on to talking with a doctor or pharmacist about what supplements are safe for you to use. You should only consider what is beneficial for your development.

If you don't have a good quality blender, I would highly suggest you get one.

Next, you need to stack up on any supplements needed and go grocery shopping with your new meal in mind. It's going to take some time to work out what you need to cook and how you can most effectively achieve your macros, but it's a fun process. Using tons of free online resources, discuss everything from the best Tupperware for meal prepping and storage to the best protein shake recipes. You won't have any problems with finding suitable material.

BOTTOM LINE

Not only do we want to streamline your nutrition so that it more effectively gets you sufficient gains, but we need food to be a way through which you can improve your health. Suppose you can healthily manage your food. In that case, there is a high possibility that you can reduce your medical problems, reduce your dependency on medications, and maintain a healthy body simply through diet and exercise.

If you haven't been eating right in the past, then understand that progress in the gym will be severely limited until you sort problems out in the kitchen first. You must develop a healthy eating routine and fuel your body with small, highly nutritious meals throughout the day, complemented with some supplements and protein shakes. Once you get into this rhythm, you will feel more robust, sleep better, and the overall physical performance of your body will improve dramatically.

3

BREAKING DOWN AND BUILDING UP YOUR BODY – INTENSITY, RECOVERY, AND WORKOUT PLANNING

STAYING TRUE

The perspective you hold shapes your reality.

The exercises that we use for strength training and many other forms of exercise are founded on a standard set of principles. These principles dictate that the movement should provide enough resistance to shock/break down the muscles. The body should then be fueled with the proper nutrition to provide the building blocks to help the muscle grow back together bigger and stronger. Finally, the body needs to rest for regrowth to occur.

Through research and experience, we have found that short explosive workouts will induce more significant gains in strength and hypertrophy. Also, some have found shorter workouts to be more engaging.

Nowhere in this philosophy is there a mention that people only between the ages of 18 and 24 should use these basic principles. Nor does it say that people near 50 and above should slow down their workouts, use alternative forms of exercise, or not expect to see gains the same way a younger athlete would.

The point of consulting with doctors and professional trainers, or even reading a book of this nature, is not to find an alternative to strength training at age 45 and beyond; it's to learn how to strength train properly, given the change in circumstances.

While the principles of strength training remain the same, the way we implement them changes. We will be discussing this equation in this chapter together with a couple of other critical topics for good physical development.

A Familiar Path

I'd also like to state that there is no need to change the exercises you do, aside from a few alterations. There are a few staple exercises that every strength athlete has to master, whether you are training for personal fitness or you want to compete in an international lifting competition.

You have to go through all four bases to make a home run, regardless of where you hit the ball.

If you think that equipment, a gym, or any external factor is limiting, I would highly suggest you brush up on the basic bodyweight exercises. If you aren't knowledgeable on these, I suggest you look at the first book in this series, as it goes into great detail about bodyweight movements. Using those simple exercises, you can get a lot more out of a workout than you would, even with a membership at your local gym. The way you train is what makes all the difference, not where you train or who you train with. Using some of the tips and tricks in this chapter, you can use those bodyweight exercises to create a routine that is easily an intermediate to an advanced level workout.

TESTOSTERONE

You've probably heard a lot about this hormone. It gets spoken about many times. Some people state it as the most crucial part of building muscle, and others may argue that it's not as important as they say. The fact of the matter is, we all have it, and we can benefit from it, especially as strength athletes.

Let me get you up to speed about why this is important.

First of all, testosterone is critical for both men and women, though it's predominantly found in higher quantities with men. However, testosterone is responsible for several physical traits and having adequate storage is vital throughout your life.

While this is generally associated with libido or sexual desire, this hormone affects far more than that. For instance, testosterone is a critical component in hair growth, skin quality, and even bone density. This hormone can even influence our mental development, our behavior, and our cognitive processes. To think that one hormone can have this impact is remarkable.

However, the fantastic ability to influence muscle development, muscle mass storage, strength, recovery, bone density, and fat burning are essential to athletes.

Sarcopenia

Like many other things in the body, testosterone production also gradually decreases with age. This hormone has a notable impact on muscle and strength development, so a decrease in testosterone production naturally leads to loss of muscle mass, a condition also known as sarcopenia. This condition is an unavoidable consequence of aging. Men and women over the age of 30 can expect to lose about 3%-8% of total muscle mass every ten years. While this may not sound like a large amount, the result can be quite dramatic when you factor in the sedentary life that most people follow. This process significantly increases the possibility of injury in later years because their bodies are weaker. As we enter the final 20 years of our lives, people find it harder to stabilize, perform daily activities, and maintain overall health. Don't worry; you still have years before the effects are noticeable, and most people between 50-60 still perform well, which gives you plenty of time to prepare and delay this process.

The Solution

Luckily, there are many things we can do to counter this natural decrease in testosterone production.

First and foremost is protein. Simply consuming enough protein can help older men retain more muscle mass. In the case of a person who is actively training, they need not only consume enough to maintain; they need to consume enough to assist muscle recovery and growth.

As we mentioned in the previous chapter, the recommended RDA is not enough for older adults. One of the main reasons for this is anabolic resistance. As the body ages, its ability to break down and synthesize protein reduces significantly. To overcome this problem, you need to eat more than the recommended daily protein intake. This is why having 0.8 to 0.9 grams of protein per pound of body weight can be very helpful in retaining the muscle mass you have. It can be challenging to eat that much protein from whole food sources such as meat and eggs, which is why it can be beneficial to add in a couple of protein shakes that can quickly help you get 70-100 grams of protein.

Furthermore, to maximize recovery and growth, it can be highly effective to consume a drink or a meal after a workout with a carbohydrate to protein ratio of 3 to 1. So a bowl of Greek yogurt that offers around 10 grams of protein and 30 grams of carbs is an excellent choice. You could also add oatmeal or other high-carb foods to a protein shake after a workout to create a drink that uses this same ratio. Moreover, this needs to be consumed within thirty minutes of completing the workout for maximum results.

Progressive Resistance Training (PRT) is the other approach to making maximum gains and helping the body use the protein that we feed it. That is to increase the resistance in a training session or through the course of a workout protocol to make maximum gains. PRT is a training technique used in many variations, though the core concept remains the same.

A thorough PRT program is all about performing the exercises correctly, increasing load, increasing repetitions, modifying rest periods, and making the workout as intense as possible without overwhelming the trainee.

A typical PRT session will include 8-10 exercises that work all the major muscle groups, starting with 12-15 rep sets. Further on, we will come back to PRT and how we get the most out of it.

An External Boost In Testosterone?

In the previous chapter, we covered how you can use various supplements to make maximum gains. Among the many supplements out there are also testosterone supplements. However, this is something I would consider avoiding.

Even though athletes use these and are renowned as a beneficial supplement, it has many side effects, most of which irreversibly impact the body. People have seen an increase in muscle mass with the use of testosterone supplements. However, fueling your body externally with synthetic hormones, whether it's growth hormones or testosterone, can seriously impact your body's ability to produce hormones. There have also been studies to suggest it can damage your body's organs and tissue.

Therefore, it is best to use dietary supplements and things that will not interfere with the natural production of hormones.

Intensity

At the core of the PRT program is intensity. How much resistance you can handle in the PRT workout, and how intense you can make the workouts.

However, it's essential to highlight the differences between power and strength. Even though I use these terms relatively interchangeably, their implications can be drastically different. Especially in the context of training and fitness sciences, these are two very distinct things.

Strength is what we train to enhance our lifting capacity. If you can bench 250 pounds with maximum effort, then if I could help you get that number up to 300, that would be considered an increase in muscle strength.

Power, on the other hand, is how effectively you can use strength in daily life. It is more reflected in how fast you can move, your flexibility, and how explosive your movements are.

While gaining strength is a primary objective, making the most of this strength is also something you should be aiming for. You want to have a solid functional physique that is not only going to help you set PRs in the gym but is also going to improve your physical capability and give you a better quality of life. In particular, it can be considerably beneficial in generating explosive power, such as your ability to quickly jump up a flight of stairs or make quick maneuvers without losing your breath. These are things that rely on the overall conditioning of your body and the state of soft tissue.

Durability

With the correct training protocol, you can expect to see exponential gains in your cardiovascular health. As we discussed in the first chapter, cardiovascular health is also essential to strength training, and if you have any severe heart-related problems, you need to take it easy with strength training.

If you want to lose weight, strength training can help you achieve that goal much faster. Although it is widely accepted that jogging burns more calories than weight training, the latter is far more likely to keep your metabolism elevated for a more extended period.

Research has shown intense workout sessions to increase an athlete's metabolism for up to 48 hours after the workout session. Meaning for up to two days after the workout, you are burning more calories than you otherwise would doing the same day-to-day tasks.

If you can complement this with fasted cardio in the morning or on days when you aren't hitting the weights, you could see some incredible results in terms of fat loss.

As we age, our joints and bones also tend to get weaker and struggle with activities such as running, hiking, or any other high-impact activities. In addition, if a person were to fall and hurt a joint or a bone, it becomes a bit more challenging to recover from such an injury at an older age. This is where strength training shines, especially when it is combined with PRT. It is a system that involves very calculated movements, reduces the stress on the body, has a meager chance of injury, and can even improve joint health.

Despite all this, strength training doesn't have to be a very time-consuming task. On the contrary, effective programs are usually short, explosive workouts that only need to be done 2 or 3 times a week to get the best results. I'm here to tell you; you don't have to work out every single day of your life. It's unnecessary, and anyone who tells you differently doesn't understand the busy lives we all lead. On the days you have a training session, you are only investing a short amount of time in enjoyable activities that will help you make consistent progress in muscle mass and body condition. So if you are on a tight schedule, strength training is the way to go.

HIGH-INTENSITY EXERCISES

You may have heard of High-Intensity Interval Training (HIIT). While that is a fantastic protocol that we will look at in more detail later, I am talking about something different here.

Using the fundamental exercises you are currently familiar with - the ones covered in the previous book, we can modify our training approach to increase the intensity of a given workout.

For instance, whether you are training a particular muscle or a full-body training day, these are a few things you can do to significantly increase the intensity of the workout.

1. More Reps In The Same Amount Of Time

This method requires you to time your workout, so if it's taking you 120 seconds to do 15 reps of a certain exercise, you want to try reaching 20 or 25 in the same 120-second window. To achieve this, you might need to lower the weight slightly, but overall, you will be getting more muscle stimulation. It's also a good idea to see how many reps you can do with a specific weight to set a benchmark for yourself. Most of us tend to focus on the number of reps rather than the time it takes to perform them, so taking a different approach to your training could spice things up and give you fresh motivation. Although, try not to forget about your form when using this method of exercise.

2. More Sets Within The Same Time

This can be a great way to energize an otherwise slow and tedious working routine. Again, you can apply this to any workout; if you manage to do three sets of 5 different exercises in a 45-minute workout, you could aim to do four sets of each the next time around. Prepare yourself because this will be far more challenging, especially if you are doing a wide variety of exercises. Overall, I'm sure your goal at this point is to be as effective as you can in your workout session, no matter how short or long it may be, in which case you should consider this.

3. More Reps In The Same Number Of Sets

This is not a time-based strategy, but the end goal is to get more work done during a workout, just like the other methods. I'm sure this doesn't need much explanation, but for example, if you do 5 sets with 12 reps each, that works out to a total of 60 reps. You could aim to do a total of 70 reps in 5. A slight adjustment, but it will go a long way, and I guarantee you will feel the difference. Near the end of your workout, consider dropping the resistance down and performing a final set to failure. This is an excellent way of building endurance.

4. Lower Rest Period Between Sets

A strategy that resonates most with the HIIT ideology, the basis of this workout is to create a circuit of exercises and complete the course with minimal rest between exercises. I know some people in the gym tend to enjoy a relaxing 5-minute rest between sets. It sounds comfortable, right? Well, unfortunately, those people aren't increasing hypertrophy at the speed that I know you'd like. Although a 3-5 minute break would absolutely help with building strength and power, a measly 30 to 90-second rest would be ideal for building muscle. Once you complete the circuit, allow yourself some recovery time with a 3-5 minute rest before it's go-time again.

The strange thing is, HIIT workouts are not something you often find in gyms; maybe people are just lazy, or perhaps they are afraid to try something different, but luckily, you're not like that. It can be highly beneficial for overall fitness, especially if fat loss is your goal. Remember when we talked about having an elevated metabolism for hours after a workout? Well, HIIT is phenomenal at that.

RECOVERY

Recovery and nutrition are the two most underrated parts of training in all sport. Though when it comes to strength training, they play a pivotal role in the kind of progress you can look to make and your body's overall wellness. Proper recovery and post-workout routines help minimize the chances of injury and prepare your body to pursue strength training for several years to come. If you want longevity in your training, then pay attention to your recovery protocol.

More and more athletes from all walks of life are learning the benefits of ice baths, stretching, foam rolling, and the many other rest and recovery systems out there. Though, I would like to draw your attention to the most effective form of recovery, sleep.

One of the biggest mistakes people make is not taking enough time to let their bodies heal, which is due to fear of losing out and slowing progression. Just getting enough shut-eye plays a massive role in how well you can recover from all the previous day's hardships, especially if you want to make the most progress possible in the least amount of time. I, myself, have fallen victim to this belief in the past. Not long ago, I fractured my ankle. At the time, I was training hard and getting into a real stride; however, my body warn down, but I ignored it because I didn't want to lose any progress. Then, at the end of an enjoyable spar fight with my teammate, I remember moving backward to evade an incoming strike and then collapsing to the floor after hearing a loud crack on my ankle. It annoyed me how something as insignificant as bouncing my foot on the mat would cause my ankle to snap, but it shows how weak humans are without sufficient rest.

You need to get between 6 - 8 hours of sleep every night, and more importantly, it would be ideal if you kept the same sleep cycle throughout the entire week. I know life isn't perfect, and sometimes you don't end up getting to bed till 1'oclock in the morning, but I urge you to try and make it a priority when you can. If your life is such that you work at night or prefer to sleep during the day, that's fine, but the hours of rest and the time you rest need to be kept as consistent as possible. Regardless of training, you will notice that your life will improve as a whole. You will experience having more energy throughout the day, focusing better, working harder, and a whole list of other physiological benefits.

Real progress and growth are made with sleep and mental evaluation, regardless of any age you may find yourself in. So the more intense your workouts, the more time you will need to recover, and I regret to say this, but there are no shortcuts.

WORKOUT PLANNING

As we previously mentioned, you need to put together a program that will work effectively for you. That is only going to be half the battle, though. Integrating it into your daily schedule and staying consistent with the program over an extended time frame is the real challenge.

It would help if you had something that considers your personal life, professional commitments, training routine, and personal preference in managing all of these things. The only way to create an excellent routine is to look at your life through a magnifying glass and figure out how to prioritize the most important things to get the most out of them and become the best version of yourself.

Moreover, it's great that you put together a plan and have made time for everything, but there will be times when something unexpected happens; the car doesn't start, or the kids need you for something that will take away your training time. This is when you need to prioritize your fitness goals and evaluate what you need to do. I don't mean that you have to take time away from what is important to you, but I suggest you make up for this lost time later. It's the same for me writing this book; even though it gets tiring sometimes and breaks consist of coffee and power naps, I know that I'm going to be happy at the end of it all.

ACTION PLAN

The best way to prepare for those unexpected moments is to get skilled in the art of adaption and compromise. So how do we do this? The best way is to build a routine that requires minimal variables: exercises with little equipment or preparation. That is why you must affirm yourself with bodyweight and resistance band training. If you are unfamiliar with these exercises, I suggest you go back and read through the chapters on bodyweight and resistance band training in The Seven Keys To Strength Training For Men Over 50. As a woman reading this, you may be thinking this book doesn't apply to you, but there is valuable information inside that you could greatly benefit from. These bodyweight exercises are something that can be performed anywhere, anytime. You don't need to rely on equipment. All you need is your body and the willingness to train. Later on, in this book, we will go through some advanced bodyweight techniques so you will have no excuses for lack of time.

However, suppose you are well versed in bodyweight training and want that extra boost in your training. In that case, you can ramp up the resistance on those exercises simply by incorporating the higher intensity ideas we have covered in this chapter. If you want to join a gym, that's great, but don't let that be an excuse not to train. Calisthenics eliminates all excuses.

BOTTOM LINE

In closing this chapter, I hope you can take away two crucial points: sufficient recovery is always necessary and progressive overloading is how you gain. And let's not forget that it doesn't have to be a time-consuming process. Even a short 20-minute workout using only bodyweight exercises with high intensity will keep you on the right track during those busy times.

4

ADVANCED BODY WEIGHT STRENGTH TRAINING

THE LEVEL BEFORE "THE NEXT LEVEL"

B asic exercises are great, especially when combined with high-intensity techniques. Still, if you want to take your physical development to the next level using minimal gear, then you are in the right place.

This chapter will cover how you can make maximum progress using as little gear as possible through advanced bodyweight exercises.

One of the most reliable ways to quickly and safely transition to these more advanced techniques is to start by simply adding intensity techniques as a filler to your standard routine. When you feel like you have 'plateaued' with muscle growth on the current workout, you can consider diving into these more advanced techniques.

A significant side effect of adding high-intensity techniques to weight training is that it supplies you with a taste of cardio. These workouts will give you a pretty heavy cardio workout. Those who focus solely on strength training may sometimes find that you run out of breath before your muscles reach fatigue. A concerning thought, no doubt, but not to worry, your cardiovascular system will soon catch up. These intense workouts will help you generate a heart rate equivalent to or even exceeding what you would otherwise attain during a short sprint. Combined with the fact that they exert a lot of pressure on all areas of your body, you will find these exercises to be quite taxing. If you are ready to incorporate more variety and even more intensity into your workout, let's get into some advanced bodyweight exercises.

LEARNING NEW BODYWEIGHT ROUTINES

Before we get started, it's essential to keep in mind that you shouldn't overexert yourself with these new exercises. While they may seem simple as you read on, they take some practice before you can execute them flawlessly.

YOUR BEST BODY AFTER 45 | 81

It would help if you took the time to properly study how the movements work as you don't want to learn them incorrectly and end up injuring yourself. Unfortunately, this book doesn't come with insurance. I have seen countless people who have injured themselves and been left with long-term health implications due to performing an exercise incorrectly. It rarely happens the first time, but if you continuously put your joints in compromising positions, they will weaken over time.

Similarly, some of these exercises are very explosive. They isolate targeted muscles to give you maximum activation. Others place an incredible amount of strain on specific muscle groups, unlike the more well-known bodyweight exercises that act more as compound movements, activating multiple muscle groups at once. In effect, when you perform several sets in succession, you entirely exhaust that muscle. Ironically, this means you are at a higher risk of being injured.

For instance, the pike press-up that targets your shoulders and upper back is often very challenging for people to perform because of the balance it requires. If you haven't spent time working on your core strength and balance, this can be difficult to execute correctly.

Before you get into exercises such as the pike press-up or the spider man press-up, you need to make sure the body is warmed up. These movements are very different from what your body is accustomed to and may require higher levels of coordination.

So, let's start with one of the most underrated body-weight exercises of all.

Pull-Ups

When it comes to measuring upper body strength, most people will emphasize how much they can bench. Some people will say lifting equal to your body is good enough, while more competitive strength athletes aim to bench twice or even three times their body weight. There is no doubt that the bench press is a challenging exercise, but it is not a complete representation of upper body strength. It predominantly focuses on the chest and the triceps, and these are only two groups among the many others in the upper body.

Okay, so I know I said earlier that most of the exercises we discussed would focus mainly on isolation exercises. Nevertheless, pull-ups and other variations are an exception due to their level of difficulty.

The fascinating part about the pull-up is it could save your life one day. For instance, if you slipped off the edge of a cliff and had to pull yourself up. Someone who couldn't perform a pull-up in the gym would perish; granted, this scenario doesn't happen in life very often, but as the saying goes - you're better safe than sorry.

The pull-up relies on nearly every muscle in your arms, your back, and even your core. It is a true test of upper body strength. Moreover, just a slight change in the pull-up movement can modify the impact of the exercise and target a different group of muscles altogether.

When working with people who are new to exercising or even those lifting weights in the gym for years, I have noticed that the pull-up is something people usually fail to utilize. Even guys with a strong bench can't always do a complete set of pull-ups.

THE ROAD TO PULL-UPS

I understand that performing consecutive pull-ups can be challenging, especially if you are on the heavy side, so my advice is to make your pull-ups a priority and do them at the start of a workout when your body is fresh. In addition to this tip, here are a few things you can do to improve pull-up strength.

1. Wide-Grip Lat Pull Downs

I If you are currently training at a gym and want to improve your pull-ups, then the lat pull-down machine will be your best friend. If you have a machine at home that can help you replicate the pull-down movement, then use that. The point is that you want to simulate the pull-up movement with weights lower than your current body weight to build upon those muscles required for a successful pull-up.

Ideally, you want to stick to the wide grip pull-downs. Although you could use close grips and other forms of pull downs, wide grips will help you train those muscles for the pull-up most efficiently. Lastly, I suggest you use a combination of low and high reps with different weights to mix things up and build your overall strength. Start with heavier weights and work your way down as your muscles start to fatigue.

2. Cable Face Pulls

Regarding workload, you will be using the same high-rep and low-rep strategy that I recommended with the wide grip pull-downs. Not only will cable face pulls improve your posture from hours of sitting at a desk, but it's also going to help you perfect your shoulder blade retraction, which is key to a good pull-up. Without proper shoulder blade movement, you can't get the real benefits of a pull-up.

3. Negative Pull-Ups

Did you know your muscles are stronger in the eccentric motion than in the concentric motion? I assume not because you're probably thinking, what the hell is this guy talking about. Well, let me put it like this; you can usually lower weights easier than lifting them. In other words, if you eliminate the lifting in the movement, it makes the exercise a lot more achievable for those who struggle, and we still get the benefits of building those muscles. Problem solved!

This is why it helps for you to train negative pull-ups. The only thing that changes with this technique is the starting position. So, to get to where your chin meets the bar, you can use a chair or a box and jump into place, with caution, of course. Then slowly lower yourself down, taking about 3-5 seconds before your arms are fully extended.

4. Lower Body

I would die a happy man if people stopped dangling their legs when they performed a pull-up. It misses out on so much opportunity because your body essentially becomes a massive lever, and where there are levers, there's resistance. Use this time to activate muscles in your core and legs. More specifically, tightening your glutes and stiffening your legs during the entire movement will help tremendously with increasing difficulty and recruiting as much muscle fiber as possible.

PERFORMING THE PERFECT PULL UP

You may already be aware of the mechanics for this exercise but let's take this time to refresh your memory.

Classic Pull Up

Start by gripping the bar slightly wider than shoulder-width with an over-the-bar grip, so your palms face away from you. Your body should remain straight in your starting position, with your arms stretched out and your legs locked in place (not dangling). From this position, you want to start pulling yourself up in a straight line till your chin is over the bar, squeezing your lats at the top and holding for one second before beginning your descent. Lower yourself gradually at a constant pace in control of your whole body. You can also cross your legs at the ankles to improve core stability. Do not attempt to swing or use momentum throughout the movement if you want to make the most of it.

Wide Grip Pull Up

As the name suggests, you will be using the exact grip you would use for a wide grip lat pull-down in this form of a pull-up. Depending on whether your arms are a weak point or not, you may find this slightly easier than the classic pull-up, though most people find it more challenging. The movement pattern remains the same as the traditional pull-up, and you can still cross your legs to stabilize the core; however, this form reduces the inclusion of the arms and isolates your back further. Another critical note would be to refrain from hoisting yourself up when your back gets fatigued. I believe it's better to do half a rep at the point of failure than complete the rep using improper technique. Another reason you should include this exercise near the beginning of a workout is to minimalize muscle fatigue.

Narrow Grip Pull Ups

I'm sure you can guess, but these are the opposite of wide-grip pull-ups. Instead of isolating your back, they rely on your arms and specifically your biceps. If you are looking for a bodyweight exercise that will work on your arms, this is the one to do.

Pull Up With Leg Raise

In this pull-up, you will be performing it exactly as you would the classic pull-up, with the difference being you tighten your core and lift your legs to form a 90-degree angle at the hip. Ensure that your body remains rigid and lower your legs before returning to the starting position. You will be tempted to swing your legs, but the more you can eliminate swing and the more precisely you can perform the activity, the more beneficial it will be.

Weighted Pull Up

As you get more comfortable with pull-ups and perform complete sets with good form, you can increase the amount of resistance throughout the movement to keep the momentum of your muscle progression. Just like a shark in the water, you have to keep moving forward. There are two main ways you can increase resistance in a pull-up; strapping a chosen weight to it or wearing a weighted vest during the exercise. The benefit of this is it gives you the freedom to decide how much resistance is suitable for you instead of relying on the weight of your body. As with all exercises, the purpose is to increase the resistance over time gradually. You can take this to the next level by doing a pause rep at the top of the movement, where you hold your chin above the bar for a count of 3 before lowering yourself back down. Nevertheless, you can hold yourself up for longer during the pause rep, but generally, a count of 3 is good if you plan on doing several sets with this pull-up routine.

Towel Grip Pull Up

If you are looking for the ultimate test of pull-up strength, then towel pull up should be your target. In this exercise the form is the same as the classic pull up however the main difference is that you are going to throw two towels over the bar where you would usually hold it with your hands and rather than holding the bar you are going to grip the part of the towel that is hanging down and then perform a pull up gripping the towels. This is a very taxing exercise as it requires you to have very solid grip strength and plenty of arm strength. Moreover, it works on your core, your back, and every other muscle that is related as it changes the grip and requires you to have really good stability to perform this movement well.

As you can see, there are many variations to the humble pull-up. You can use it in numerous ways to get the most out of your workout. If you can master the various pull-up types, you can get an incredibly strenuous, complete upper body workout. So, I urge you not to let this opportunity go to waste.

ADVANCED BODY WEIGHT EXERCISES

Before I begin listing off exercises for you, let me emphasize that you may already have an understanding of some or even all of the activities in this book. However, my goal is not to teach you every new movement; it's to show you how to perform them with perfect form and precision. So please take some time to read over the exercises you already know to ensure everything is done correctly.

Let's get into some more advanced techniques that will help you take your training to the next level and add some diversity to your workouts.

The Scissor V-Up

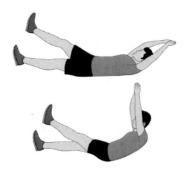

If you find that crunches aren't challenging enough, this will be perfect for you. The movement may appear confusing at first, but once you grasp the rhythm of the exercise, it will be exceptional at activating the rectus abdominis. As the name suggests, this movement combines the V-up with scissor kicks; all we are doing is putting the two together.

1. We begin laying on our back with our elbows

out and our hands touching the side of our head (not holding behind it).

2. From here, I'd like you to raise both legs slightly and start pumping out scissor kicks.

3. Now, simultaneously raise your upper body using your core and crunch. You don't have to place too much emphasis on the movement of your upper body; simply raising to a 120-degree angle with the floor and then back down again is sufficient.

4. It is considered one rep when your upper body comes back to the starting position. However, the legs should be in constant motion until you finish the set.

Dragon Walk

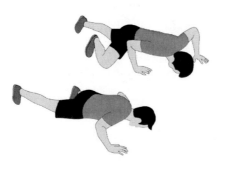

Think of this exercise as a walking push-up. You will need more room for this exercise as it is not something you can do in a small area. Your backyard would be great or any other open space where you can move freely and measure distance.

1. We begin in the top push-up position.
2. Bring your left elbow backward and bring your left knee forward till they meet. So, one side of your body should be crunched together with one elbow and knee touching each other, and the other side spread out.
3. Now, as your elbow and knee meet, lower yourself as you would with a regular push-up.
4. As you come up, lift your hand and move it forward slightly. Then, alternate to the other side and repeat the process, moving in a straight line.

The dragon walk can be a little challenging to master at first, but it's a great way to train your chest and your legs to a lesser degree once you get the hang of it.

Jumping Lunges

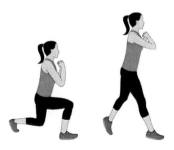

This is a more explosive variation of the lunge that forces you to possess a greater balance. This subsequently strengthens the smaller muscles and tendons in the legs, an excellent exercise for building stability in the lower half of your body. Let's go through it.

1. Stand straight with your feet shoulder-width apart and your head looking in front of you.
2. Take a step forward and lower yourself until you make a 90-degree angle at the knee. Ensure your heel is glued to the floor for the front leg. Remember to keep your core tight throughout the movement and have your hips facing forward.
3. Now, rather than just stepping back into the

starting position, drive your body into the air and switch legs, so you land with the opposite stance. You don't need to jump high for this to be effective, so instead, focus on landing softly and maintaining balance.

Pike Roll Out

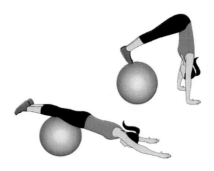

For this, you will need a fitness ball, preferably a large one, as it won't be as effective if you can't get enough altitude. This one may sound pretty confusing because the movement is reasonably odd but try your best to understand, and don't forget to use the illustrations for reference.

1. You will start in a push-up position with the

ball underneath you and your shins laying on top of it.

2. The ball should sit no higher than your knees, so you have plenty of room to roll rather than keeping it by your thighs, limiting your range of motion.

3. In the push-up position, I want you to tighten your core muscles and roll the ball up while bending out at the hips until the center of the ball is against your feet.

4. At this point, your upper body should nearly be in the handstand position. Now I want you to push out so that the ball starts moving up your legs again.

5. Continue to push your body back further so that the ball continues to roll up your calves and onto your quads. Your arms should be completely stretched out at the end of the movement and the ball underneath your thighs.

6. To complete this exercise, slowly roll back to the starting push-up position.

7. The pike rollout is probably one of the best exercises for activating the entire core, and because of this, it requires a lot of energy. If you cannot manage a complete a full set, it's okay to stop after a few reps before continuing the set.

Frozen V Sit

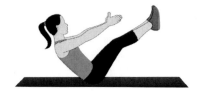

The V sit is a fantastic exercise for seasoned trainees due to its high difficulty. It targets muscles such as the rectos abdominis, internal and external obliques, and hip flexors. This exercise is perfect if you enjoy cycling because it builds the muscles that help elevate your legs up to your hip. However, please take caution if you experience back pain; this isometric movement puts pressure on the spine and can do more harm than good if you already suffer from back pain. If this is the case for you, I advise leaving this exercise out of your ab routine.

1. Lay flat on the ground with your arms to your side and your legs flat on the floor.
2. You will start off doing a crunch with your

upper body while simultaneously lifting your legs. Keep your legs straight and bring your upper and lower body together to form the V shape.

3. You should be balancing on your gluteus maximus/hip, wherever feels the most comfortable. I also suggest stretching your arms out parallel with the floor for extra balance.

4. Try to hold this position for a total of 30 seconds to test the water.

Before moving on, I have a few tips that might come in handy with the V sit. The first being to bend your legs at the knee if you are experiencing pain in your back; this can decrease the pressure on your spine. The second tip is to bring your body up to make the exercise easier and lean back to make it harder, giving you a lot of customization with this movement.

One-Legged Burpees

This burpee variation allows you to isolate one leg and get a more intense workout on each leg. I know for a fact, you will be feeling the burn on this one, no matter who you are.

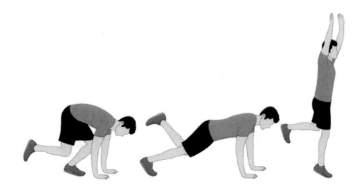

1. Begin in a standing position and lift one foot off the floor.
2. Lower yourself onto the ground by squatting on that leg and falling into a push-up position. Your other leg should remain off the floor throughout.
3. Then, perform a push-up with one leg before bringing your hands to your feet and rising again.
4. Drive up with your leg and jump at the end, landing on the same leg and going back into the push-up position to repeat the process, or alternate and switch legs at that point.

In this exercise, it's best to completely exhaust one leg and then perform the exercise with the other leg, but if you find yourself struggling, you can alternate.

Power Push-Ups

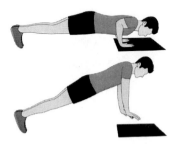

Power push-ups take it to the next level by incorporating more speed and more explosive power in every rep. While there isn't a big difference, you will notice that it is incredibly more challenging to complete a set.

1. Unlike a standard push-up, you begin in the second half of the movement, with your body lowered. This is your starting position.
2. Drive your body up with enough force to lift your hands just above the ground.
3. Your hand positioning should remain the same as you catch yourself. However, instead of

landing and stopping the forces pulling you down, I want to use that momentum to ease into another rep. This way, we can prevent any damage your joints would take from the impact.

ACTION PLAN

Now that you have gone through these exercises, you can incorporate the ones that most appeal to you. If you aren't currently doing pull-ups, chin-ups, or any variation, I highly recommend you add these into your workouts. For someone who has no experience doing these exercises, likely, you will not be able to perform them perfectly in succession, but don't let that discourage you; it's only natural.

Work your way up slowly to understand each movement till you can perform several reps safely and without chance of injury.

If you are more interested in moving weights in the gym, or perhaps you dabble in various equipment at home, then get your barbells ready and let's swiftly move on to our next chapter.

5

CRANKING IT UP – GETTING INTO FULL BODY WORKOUTS IN THE GYM

THE WEIGHT ROOM

Although bodyweight exercises are practical and easily manageable, they don't quite hit the spot, in my opinion. There is something to moving iron that changes your whole outlook towards strength training. Getting that sense of achievement when you go up in weight gives me satisfaction every single time. Maybe it's because of the gym's energy; perhaps it's because we have been taught through a widespread belief that the gym is where great bodies and athletes are built. Maybe the reason is simple; humans have been drawn to tools since the day we learned how to use them. I'm sure we could have continued to live as a species with no access to aids other than our hands, but we chose to expand our capabilities as humans. It's the same with resistance training; we could restrict ourselves to bodyweight training... but what's the fun in that!

I'm sure most of you can agree that having some equipment adds variety and entertainment to your workout, whether you are using free weights or machines. Doing the same routine of bodyweight squats and pulls ups does have its advantages, but what is the point of devoting your life to something you get no joy out of, especially in a world where most of us spend hours at work in a job we don't like. For many people, bodyweight training will be their second priority, something they do when they don't have the time or the facilities. Nevertheless, their preference is to get into the weight room and work with the tools they love.

Whether at home or a shared space, a gym is a fantastic approach to physical fitness and strength development; however, the vast pit of information out there can get overwhelming at times. Not to mention the "bro-science" and the fact that most of the information you will find online is just a subjective narrative of someone with few real credentials to back up their claims.

How will you know who you can trust and what you should be doing?

This chapter will break down everything you need to know in creating a workout that works for you. Hopefully, this will allow you to make decisions based on knowledge and not have to rely on a program you don't fully understand.

Let's get into it.

Optimum Weight Training

I want you to start on a blank slate. For now, I want you to try and let go of any beliefs, ideas, or notions you have about resistance training. Please don't take offense to this remark as I'm not saying that anything you already know is wrong; I'm saying that you can't put more water in a cup when it's already full.

Aside from the standard run-of-the-mill machinery you see in the gym, there is equipment that most people are entirely unaware of; you would be surprised how innovative the industry has become. For instance, the reverse-hyper machine was invented and manufactured by the infamous Louie Simmons of West coast Barbell. This incredible machine has helped victims of lower back pains for years, from the average 50-year old who has spent 30 years behind a desk to an elite powerlifter who damaged his spine after a 1100 pound squat. The fundamental principles behind this engineering masterpiece include allowing someone to train their lower back without weights that can potentially over-load your spine while still creating resistance. Although not found in many gyms today, this is a worthy investment if you have the money. With the right machinery and the proper knowledge, your gym can be the workshop where you build the perfect body and amend any damage.

You can get some tremendous results by just doing a 30-minute workout three times a week. However, you need to be consistent if you want to see any meaningful results.

I believe you should give yourself at least three months before you jump to a conclusion with any workout. Anyone trying to develop an evaluation of the effectiveness of a movement before the three-month mark would be ludicrous. With any given exercise or workout routine, it takes months to see a noticeable difference in hypertrophy. That is why it is impossible to rate an activity beforehand. The only exception would be if the exercise were causing pain, and in that case, you should consider seeking other methods.

Secondly, I'd like to remind you that no exercise on earth is valuable without using perfect form consistently. This is 100 times more evident now as a trainee with experience. For a complete beginner, the muscles will still get some stimulation from using the improper form. However, once your muscles build up a tolerance to regular stress, they require a concentrated force to help break them down again, and the best way is through perfect form and progressive overloading. That means no more rushing through your reps and making sure every movement is controlled and precise. I'm sure you already know this, but it's easy to forget when you're fatigued.

The gym can be a social area but try to resist turning it into a get-together. I firmly believe that every gym should have a warm, friendly and energetic environment but not at the expense of a person's time. Remember, you are here to get results, not to relax. That comes after when you reek the rewards from a productive day.

The only way short workouts are going to work is if you are swift with your actions. They should be explosive and very well planned so that when you enter the gym, you don't spend the first ten minutes thinking about what you feel like doing.

You've probably noticed the massive difference in appearance between bodybuilders and powerlifters, but why is this? You generally see powerlifters with more pump to their muscles and bodybuilders with greater definition. But this is not due to genetics or drugs. In reality, the reason is primarily the exercises they choose to perform.

Let me tell you why.

COMPOUND VS. ISOLATION MOVEMENTS

Simply put, compound movements are exercises that will stimulate a large muscle group or a movement that encourages more than one muscle group—for instance, the bench press. Not only will this trigger massive stimulation in your chest, but also your arms, your core, and even your glutes have to put in some effort to get that weight off your chest.

On the other hand, isolation movements focus on a very particular area or even a single muscle. For instance, bent-over dumbbell flies are all about your rear deltoids, with a slight impact on your traps. Another example is the commonly known bicep curl that only stimulates the long head and short head of the bicep.

The only reason you should be doing isolation exercises is if you want to train a particular muscle group. Let's say if you lacked strength in your right shoulder or tried to put your efforts towards bigger arms. It will not be ideal if your goal is fat loss or gaining strength evenly throughout your body. Not to mention, it is incredibly laborious to train these tiny muscles, which can be good for growth but can also leave you unable to use those muscles in assisting another workout the following days.

On the other hand, compound exercises have a ton of benefits and few drawbacks. They are even more beneficial for older people as they are much less stressful on the body and essentially give you more bang for your buck when considering muscle activation.

Take, for example, The leg press machine - a ubiquitous piece of equipment that you will find in any decent gym, providing you with an excellent exercise for your legs. It allows you to move weight without worrying about all the form considerations of a squat. You don't need any assistance, and the risk of injury is significantly lower.

It's very calorically taxing since you are hitting such a large muscle group and engaging muscles in other parts of your body. You might not feel it right away, but the next day you will feel depleted; the reason being, your body has to spend energy repairing more muscles than it would with an isolation movement.

Suppose you have arthritis or flexibility problems that hinder your ability to perform things like squats and deadlifts. In that case, the leg press machine will hit the same muscles without the high risk of injury. In fact, the secondary muscles that assist in the lift are usually the limiting factor in movements such as the deadlift. Through machines such as the leg press machine, you can work on the main muscle groups supporting your legs to help induce hypertrophy at a similar rate.

As we discussed earlier, one of the critical elements to developing muscle size and strength is testosterone. The more testosterone you have, the better your body will build muscle. While you do get testosterone from external sources, it is a naturally occurring hormone in your body created in response to certain conditions. One of the best ways to increase testosterone production in your body is to work your larger muscles so that your body responds by producing the testosterone necessary to help in muscle regeneration. Many body-builders do squats, deadlifts, and heavy leg presses, simply for the testosterone boost. You get a lot more testosterone when you hit these bigger muscles, and the benefits of this hormone influence the entire body. Compound exercises work exceptionally well if you are a woman and lack the natural formation of testosterone in the body compared to men.

A higher level of natural testosterone will help you see results much quicker. Whether you are losing fat, gaining strength, or just looking to improve the condition of your body, testosterone is that magic hormone that does it all.

This magic hormone will also help in recovery. So doing more compound exercises will have you coming back to the gym sooner, though you might not be that willing considering how physically taxing the activity is.

However, don't be fooled by my praise of compound exercises, nothing is perfect, and that rule applies to compound movements. There are two drawbacks to consider when using this form of exercise.

1. Some muscles don't get their time in the light - You just finished a session of heavy squats, and you're feeling great because you saved time and your muscles feel sore, so you move on. In reality, most of the load was controlled by the gluteus maximus and the quadriceps; meanwhile, the calves get left out, and you never get those herculean-looking legs I know you want.

2. One weak muscle makes the whole team vulnerable - The problem with compound exercises is you don't know which muscles are lacking and which are excelling. All your body will tell you is how much it can lift with all of them combined. The only way to test their strength is to use isolation exercises and find the weakest links. After intensive work on the

weaker muscles, I guarantee your lifting power in compound exercises will increase dramatically.

So, if there are drawbacks to both types of exercise, what's the answer? The secret to maximizing your potential in the gym or at home is utilizing both. It is vital to have a mixture of both because they complement each other beautifully. Think of compound exercises as the foundations of the house that provide support and isolations exercises as the furniture that adds to the house and gives it beauty.

We often come across the phrase of hitting a plateau in training. Essentially, your body has become accustomed to the stress placed on your muscles and struggles to break past that point of exhaustion so it can rebuild.

Workouts no longer leave you with the slightly uncomfortable yet very satisfying muscle pain the next day. You don't experience the same kind of pump, and you don't see much visible growth.

The solution to this situation is to shock your muscle back into growth, either by training in a new way or putting them through stress they haven't experienced before. The best way to push past this barrier is to play around with different volumes of your current exercises in terms of weight to rep ratio. For example, if you tend to do higher reps with low resistance, switch to a lower rep workout, and vice-versa. Another easy fix is to change the exercises you are accustomed to with some new ones in hopes of triggering a reaction. I will highlight some of the best practices, so hopefully, you can take some away and incorporate them into your routine.

COMPOUND EXERCISES

In the next section, we will look at the exact exercises you can do in the gym using weights or machines to train, but before that, it is crucial to understand the philosophy behind it.

Everyone has a weak area in their body. For some, it might be their triceps. It might be their rotator cuffs for others, but there is always that one area that tends to be weaker or smaller than the rest. Most people pay less attention to their vulnerable regions or perhaps the muscles they don't enjoy exercising. This can lead to imbalances in the body.

So, the best piece of advice I can give you is to take a balanced approach and try not to neglect your weak spots for any reason.

As we will be using compound exercises, the added benefit is there is no need to divide workouts into body-part categories. I.E., Chest day, leg day, arms, etc., instead we will divide routines according to the two main sections of the body. This approach allows for more training, and accumulating research indicates that training muscle groups more than once a week can maximize hypertrophy. It is a simple and effective strategy that I suggest you employ if you haven't already.

Splits

As we are going to be using compound exercises there is no need to break things down like what bodybuilders would usually do i.e., chest day, leg day, arms, etc. instead we have divided workouts according to the two main sections of the body. This approach will work out every muscle in each section of the body and over the course of a week you will have worked out every muscle group in the body. You will be planning your weekly routine on an upper/lower split.

Upper Body

Bench Press

There are many variations for the bench press like incline bench press, decline bench press, and dumbbell bench press. However, we will be focusing on the standard flat barbell bench press that stimulates the entire chest, and to a lesser degree, the triceps and shoulders.

If you want to focus more on the triceps, switch to a close grip bench press, and for the shoulders, alternate to a wide grip. Although a common problem with people your age is shoulder discomfort while doing bench press, so to combat this, I would advise that you apply a dumbbell floor press into your routine. This will ease the pressure off the shoulder joints while building stability due to the arms working independently.

There are many variations for you to pick from, depending on your situation. So to keep things simple, I will go through the standard bench press because the core principles are mostly the same throughout all the variations.

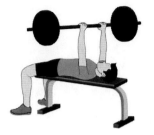 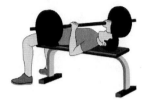

1. Start by aligning the bar with the center of the bench perfectly.
2. Lay on the bench with your eyes parallel with the bar.
3. In terms of hand placement. It can vary depending on arm length, so an excellent way to determine the best hand position for you would be to get your arms into the bench press position, with your elbows at about 75 degrees away from your body. You don't want to extend your elbows any further because it can put your rotator cuffs in jeopardy. Finally, you want to make sure your forearms are facing straight up - this is your bench press position; from here, let your hands fall back and grab onto the bar.
4. Before lifting the bar off the rack, you want to pull your shoulder blades down and slightly lift your chest, so you create a stable bass to lift. Also, make sure your feet are directly under your knees so that you can generate power from your legs.
5. Lift the bar and move it into your bench press position over your chest. From here, it's pretty simple; lower it straight down, breathe, and then up again as you exhale. If you have weak or injured shoulders, don't lower the bar all the way down to your chest before raising it again.

It's a good idea to start light in order to perfect the movement. Also, make sure the arch in your back is in your upper back and not in your mid or lower back.

Pull Over

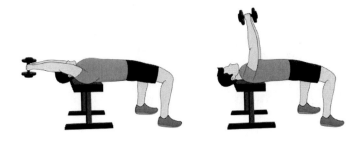

Just like squats for the lower body, the dumbbell pull-over includes every muscle group in your upper body and has become a running debate whether it's a chest or back exercise. Fortunately for you, it doesn't matter because your focus is on the entire upper body, not individual muscle groups.

1. Pick up a dumbbell and sit down right beside a bench.

2. Hold the dumbbell upright and cup the top weight with both hands.

3. Hold the dumbbell over your head and bridge up onto the bench while keeping your glutes tight.

4. The bench should be going across your upper back and shoulders and your arms reaching directly up to the ceiling. This is your starting position.

5. Now, slowly lower your arms behind you, keeping them stretched out but with a slight bend at the elbow until they are nearly horizontal with the floor. On the way down, try to take between 3-4 seconds before raising them back to the starting position.

This exercise works best with higher reps, so if you are doing 10-12 reps on other activities, try doing 16-18 reps for the pull-over. Also, start light as it can get challenging to balance the weight in your hands with this movement.

Lat Pull-Down

The Pull-down is a fantastic exercise to build back strength and muscle growth. If you cannot do multiple pull-ups on a bar, this will help you build up to that.

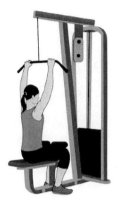 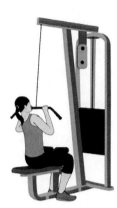

1. Grip the bar where it bends on either side. Some people prefer an open grip, but I think it's unnecessary, so I suggest using a closed grip. A general rule of thumb is that the wider your grip, the more activation you will get in your back; however, this coincidently makes it more challenging.
2. Make sure your legs are tucked tightly under the knee brace.
3. Lean back slightly and pull the bar down towards your collar bone till it is below chin level.
4. Try to avoid pulling down in front of you as it puts stress on your shoulder joints. You lean

back so it can come straight down and touch your upper chest.

You can do many variations with the pull-down, and while they all hit the back muscles, the different styles allow you to hit other areas to a degree. The standard wide grip lat pull-down is a great movement to activate the entire back.

Rows

The row is another fantastic exercise for the back that you can do in several different ways. Both the dumbbell and barbell rows are incredible for muscular hypertrophy, but I will go through the barbell row because it engages both sides of the back and allows you to pile on more weight, which leads to higher strength.

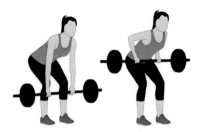

1. Unfortunately, most of us don't have the hamstring flexibility required to pick the bar up from the floor correctly, and we want to avoid curling the lower back. So, I want you to deadlift the bar into a standing position with an overhand grip if your focus is the entire back and an underhand grip if you're planning to target the lats. I would recommend having your feet at shoulder-width apart and grip the bar slightly out from your knees; however, if your goal is to target the traps and rear deltoids, then take a wider grip.

2. From the standing position, keep your back straight and push your hips out while slightly bending the knees until you reach a point where your hamstrings stop you from going any further; it's between 15-45 degrees for most people.

3. This is your starting position. From here, tighten your core and imagine lifting your elbows to the point where they create a 90-degree angle.

4. Remember to squeeze your shoulder blades together on every rep.

Barbell Shoulder Press

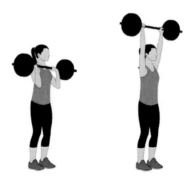

Also known as the military press, this gives you an incredible shoulder workout that also targets your back.

1. This is a relatively simple movement, but there are some key points we need to discuss when doing the shoulder press. You can start with the barbell either on the floor or on a rack (it doesn't really matter).
2. Lift the barbell off the rack into the starting position with your elbows at a 90-degree angle and your forearms directly under the bar.
3. The key to maximizing this exercise is where you place your hands. A big mistake would be maintaining a wide grip because it forces your

elbows to push back, exposing your shoulders.
Ideally, you want to place your hands no more
than shoulder-width apart when you lift.

4. Fully extend your arms before returning.

Bar Dips

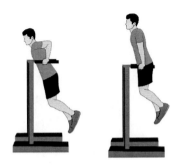

Bar dips are an excellent exercise for the arms that can
be modified with dumbbells, a weighted jacket, or even
ankle weights to increase resistance.

1. Get up on the dip machine and maintain a
   neutral position without pushing your body
   too far forward or too far back from your
   arms.
2. Lower yourself down to a 90-degree angle at
   the elbow with a neutral center of gravity. Keep

122 | BRYANT WILLIS

your elbows behind you and avoid letting them
flare out.

3. Slowly come back up to the top position and
maintain a good shoulder blade posture
throughout the movement.

The main thing to note with this movement is to resist
using your shoulders to carry your weight. Suppose the
exercise is too challenging to rely on your arms; I'd
prefer you shorten the range of motion until you
develop more strength. The next step would be the dips
with gymnastic rings; this requires tremendous
stability to perform.

Mid Portion

Many people neglect the core, but if you wish to
achieve ultimate fitness and maximize your gains, you
need to give it some love, as it helps support other
muscles for increased strength and overall gains.

Hanging Leg Raises

The hanging leg raise is often underutilized because it
requires grip strength and the support of many other
muscles. However, this movement is exceptional for
training your upper and lower abdominals, as well as
the hip flexors. It requires a lot of strength and control
to perform, so keep that in mind, and if you find your-

self struggling, switch to knee raises. The rules apply to both variations. I shall go through the three main tips to consider when performing this exercise.

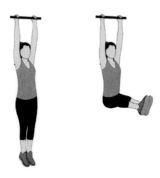

1. Keep your elbows locked and core tight at all times to avoid the temptation of recruiting other muscles.
2. Maintain a straight back, vertical with the floor throughout the entire movement.
3. Have your legs start and return slightly in front of your body to minimize the urge to swing and sustain tension on the abdominals.

Lower Body

Barbell Squat

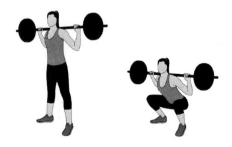

This is a mighty movement that strength athletes swear by; it does not require further introduction because we are all aware of the exercise. However, I need to cover some tips, so we are all doing it right.

This exercise does not begin at the rack. First, we must remember to warm up our shoulders sufficiently before grabbing that barbell. The reason being that some of you and myself included, experience tight shoulders, and the necessary position for barbell squatting requires us to have decent flexibility. With that said, let's get into it.

1. Start by standing with your feet shoulder-width apart and your toes pointing out for stability

while the barbell rests on your shoulders. Grip the bar a few inches away from your shoulder. Keep a closed grip or, if you prefer, an open grip with your thumbs resting underneath the bar.

2. Now, if you don't mind, I kindly ask that you do this one with a smaller weight than what you're used to because most people don't go through the full range of motion, and it can make the movement significantly harder.

3. You need to go through the full range of motion if you want to avoid acute or chronic pain in your knees. Stick your glutes out and sit down past the 90-degree bend in your knees, keeping your chin up and chest out throughout the movement. The barbel should go up and down in a straight line.

4. Your heels should stay on the floor at all times so you can push up with your heels instead of your toes.

5. When it comes to squats, you should breathe in before initiating the movement and breathe out when you return to the starting position. Resist breathing out when you are in a deep squat because it relieves tension in the core and can leave your back vulnerable.

If you find that your heels are coming up off the floor, you can put a plate under your heel and raise it a couple of inches off the ground. This should help keep your heel stable. However, remember that higher flexibility is achieved by adequately warming up and cooling down.

Leg Press

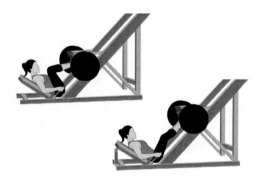

1. Get on the leg press machine and adjust the plate so that when you sit on the bench, your legs create a 90-degree angle. Lay your feet flat on the plate while keeping your back straight and holding the handles on each side.
2. Lift the plate slightly so that you can release the locks on either side.
3. With the machine unlocked, extend the weight track out till your legs are nearly straight, and

then bring it back down as far as you can without rounding your lower back. You don't want to lock your knees at extension as it can lead to injuries.

This is a great exercise that you can either do with both legs together or one leg at a time if you want to isolate it further.

Barbell Hip Thrust

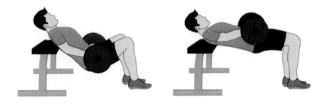

The barbell hip thrust is an exercise primarily for your glutes. If you are feeling this in your quads or lower back, you need to adjust the form. For strength training, you should keep reps low and go heavy, whereas for hypertrophy, keep the weight light and the reps high. However, if you are new to the exercise, use light weights or even just the bar to familiarize yourself with the movement.

1. Sit on the floor next to a secured bench or platform. Ideally, the bench should be resting in line with your shoulder blades. The higher the platform in relation to your back, the harder the movement.
2. Pull the barbell onto your waist just under your belly button.
3. Bring your feet in relatively close to your body.
4. From this position (holding the barbel on both sides), I want you to use your glutes to shoot your hip up in the air until you cannot comfortably go any higher and then slowly bring them down.
5. Keep the glutes tight throughout and squeeze for a second or two at the top of the movement before returning.

In these exercises, you don't want to swing the weight. It should be a very controlled movement in which your glutes are constantly engaged. Swinging will induce more knee extension and will use more quad activation. Also, swinging the weight, especially when using heavy weights, is very demanding on your lower back.

Keeping your chin tucked in, and eyes on the barbell throughout the movement will help you maintain much better spine posture and will help significantly reduce the rounding of the lower back. Tuck your tail bone in to protect your back alignment and squeeze your glutes.

Floor bridges use the same principle but can be performed without a bench. If you are doing this movement for the first time, it's a good idea to start with floor bridges to understand the action and get used to engaging your glutes. It's also a good warm-up/cooldown for a barbell hip thrust.

ISOLATION EXERCISES

As I said earlier, these exercises complement compound movements. Ideally, it would help if you pumped out your isolation exercises at the start of the workout while your muscles are fresh. It becomes harder to use muscles individually when they are exhausted, and you won't be able to get the most out of the exercise, or worse, your form will suffer.

Let's look at some of the best isolation exercises I have come across over the years.

Reverse Grip Bench Press

You've probably been doing bench presses for quite a while now. However, many people aren't familiar with what an upper chest pump feels like, and they assume if an exercise is designed for the chest, it will evenly activate the entire area. That's almost like saying bicep curls will effectively work your triceps if you do enough reps.

Recent studies have shown that a flat bench press hits the upper pecs to a lesser degree, but an incline bench press hits the upper pecs 5% more effectively. However, that is not an exceptional gain, and many would argue that you could probably get just as much upper pec stimulation from a flat bench press if you used the right training style.

If you really want to get the most gains for your upper chest, I recommend the reverse grip bench press. In studies, this bench press style has been shown to activate 30% more of the upper pecs compared to the regular flat bench press. Now that is a serious increase in muscle stimulation that will get you results guaranteed.

This is how you do it.

1. Set yourself up on a flat bench just as you

would with a regular bench press. The only difference is that rather than holding the bar with your palms facing away from you, you rotate your hands and grip the bar with your palms facing towards you.

This is a very counter-intuitive style for your muscles, and the movement can be tricky, so I suggest you keep the weights low for now. As you get more familiar with the action, you can work your way up in weight.

Cobra Forearm Curl

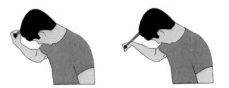

Your forearm is a small but essential muscle group. Without solid grip strength, you are severely limited in the exercises you do since most activities in the gym require you to hold the weights in your hands for extended periods. This includes the pull-up that we discussed earlier in the book.

However, there is a surprising reason why you don't want to stick to traditional forearm exercises; nearly all of them will force you to let the bar or dumbbell roll into your finger, and often, to the very tip of your fingers. Now, this might give you the illusion that you are getting more muscle activation, but in reality, you are setting yourself up for a lot of problems, not in just your fingers but also your elbows. The strain on your fingers and fingertips is one of the leading causes of elbow pain. That is why the exercise we are about to discuss offers a full range of motion in the wrist without relying on your fingers, making these movements a whole lot more effective and safer to perform.

The cobra forearm curl is a fantastic exercise that will help you build more mass on the forearms and enough grip to a one-arm pull-up if you're feeling up to it.

Here's how we do it.

1. Attach the cable handles (also known as resistance band handles) using the cable machine. Then adjust the height of the machine, so it is level with your shoulder.
2. Next, grab the handle with your palm facing away from the machine and take one big step

out to create resistance. Curl your palm forward when you are ready, keeping your forearm vertical. Try to curl your hand as far forward as possible to get the most activation.

3. Slowly release the handle as far back as your wrist will let you before returning to the starting position.

Also, if you don't have access to a gym or want to work on your forearms at home, you can do this same exercise with a band. Just secure the band to something sturdy, grip the handle in your palm and start curling those forearms.

Lying Tricep Extension

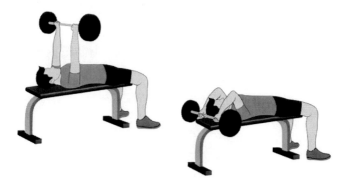

It's a great exercise that I'm sure many of you are familiar with, but let's go through it to ensure you get the most out of your workout.

1. Load up the easy bar as the pronated position of the bar will relieve stress on your wrists. with a reasonably challenging weight, place your index finger on the dents of either side and grab the bar.
2. Lay down flat on the bench and hold your arms straight above your upper chest.
3. Now, move your arms back over your face. By doing this, we apply greater force on the triceps and allow a full range of motion over the head.
4. Bend with your elbows and lower the bar while keeping everything else tight.

Moreover, the slight variation that I have described will include activation of the interior tricep; this targets the long head of the tricep, which will give you that thick arm look.

Ab Rollouts

We have all seen those little wheel contraptions somewhere before, whether in the gym or your local store. Even though they share the resemblance of a kid's toy, they are incredibly beneficial for your abs if used correctly.

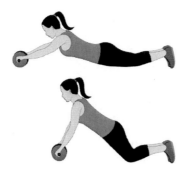

Secondly, it's not like purchasing one of these would require you to break the bank. You can grab one for ten bucks, and for a solid abdomen, I believe that is well worth the sacrifice.

Essentially, all you have to do is get down on all four, hold the handles with both hands, roll the wheel out while keeping your legs fixed and then return to the starting position.

At first glance, this is a simple exercise for beginners, and I'm sure that's why people claim to do 50 - 100 reps at a time. Well, if this is you, I'm sorry to say, but you have been doing it wrong. Follow these rules I've laid out below, and you will see the difference in difficulty skyrocket.

1. Stop bending your elbows

Bending your elbows takes nearly all the load off of your core and places it on your shoulders and triceps. Keep your arms completely straight, and then do the rollout. As the abs get tired, you will be tempted to bend your elbows; take a break in the starting position, and continue using immaculate form.

2. Pulling back with your arms

Lowering yourself into the rollout is relatively easy, but pulling yourself back is the challenging part. This is where a lot of people cheat themselves and use their arms to complete the process. You will notice this if you see your arms starting to move the roller back before your core has initiated the movement. Again, you are taking the pressure off the core and transferring it to other muscles, which is not the aim of this exercise. If you find it too challenging to pull yourself back in, reduce the distance you roll out. Start with a shorter extension, and then work your way along as you develop abdominal strength.

3. Taking a seat

One of the easiest ways to take the tension off your core, even if your arms are dead straight, is to move your hips too far. It would be best to extend your body out as far as possible, although you want to make sure you don't sit back on your hips and relieve tension on your return to the starting position. Instead, you want to keep your glutes tight and firmly ahead of your knees through the movement. The way to achieve this is by curling your back up into the air. I usually wouldn't advise flexion of the spine, but you are curling the upper back with no weight bearing down on it, so you should be fine. Try to envision an imaginary line where your hips cannot cross beyond your knees.

4. Hip stance

Speaking of the hips and where they should be, you should also understand that not only does the incorrect hip position impact the effectiveness of this exercise, but it also puts your lower spine in a precarious situation. If your hip is moving past your knees, you will notice that your lower back is flexing forwards and backward, creating a serious inward and outward curve during the movement. This is highly harmful to the lower back. Ideally, you want to be driving your hips towards your belly button throughout the movement.

This will protect our lower back in both the extension and the exercise contraction.

5. Diversity

If you have mastered all the points mentioned previously and your form is on point, then there is a step you can take to make the ab roll out more challenging. Rather than extending out in a straight line, try adding a slight turn at the end of the extension. This variation will target the core slightly differently and give you immense activation of the obliques. This workout doesn't include taking a sharp turn as soon as you launch yourself into the extension but just a slight change of direction at the end of your reach. This is less of a problem and more of a bonus to get the most out of the rollout. Alternate between directions to get an excellent core workout.

Dumbbell Goblet Abductor Lunge

We all want those crazy legs with size and vascularity, but just like the arms, you also need to target the muscles on both sides of the leg to get that complete look. Moreover, if you want balance and functional strength, you will have to work more than just your quads and hamstrings. The dumbbell goblet abductor lunge helps you do just that by targeting the hip flexors.

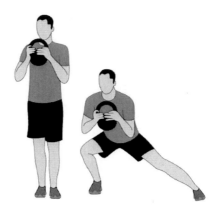

Here is how you can do it.

You want to have a smooth surface that you can slide along, preferably with socks on. You can either do this on a wooden floor or get a wall lamination sheet.

1. You will start in a standing position with a dumbbell resting between both palms and held close to your chest.
2. With this exercise, you aim to squat down with one leg and the other leg sliding out to your side.

It's also vital that you don't just stand up on your way back to the standing position; instead, you slide your way up. This is going to create the tension that you need to help those hip flexors and side abductors.

Alternate between both legs doing 10-12 reps on each leg to get a solid workout.

Calf Raises

The calf muscle is another weak point for athletes of all ages and either gender. So to counteract this, it would help if you gave them special attention at some point in your routine. I'll walk you through it.

Standing up straight, keeping good posture, lift yourself onto your toes. Hold the raised position for 2 seconds, and then lower yourself back down.

That's all there is to it, but there are a few ways that you can get more out of this exercise. Remember, the calf might be a small muscle, but they are powerful and often require more stimulation.

You can do this hanging off the edge of a box, a gym step, or even just the staircase at home to increase the range of motion.

Raise yourself up, as you would on the ground, but on the way down, let your ankle extend down till as far as your current flexibility allows. The lower your heel can go from the ball of your feet, the greater the stretch in the calves and the more resistance you will have on the way up.

If you are doing this at a gym, you could use a couple of plates to stand on as the principles remain the same. However, if you are in the gym, you will probably have access to a calf raise machine which is fantastic for this movement as it allows you to add on a lot more than just bodyweight.

If you are doing this at home and want to add more resistance, grab a few dumbbells and hold them down at your side. Another way to increase resistance at home is to do single-leg calf raises. I don't think I need to explain why using one leg is more demanding than two; however, they can be a great workout.

Generally, one calf will be slightly more robust than the other, so performing single-leg calf raises can test that theory.

ACTION PLAN

If you are looking to join a gym or invest in equipment for your home, you should start with the needed equipment for the exercises we have mentioned.

Secondly, try doing an upper/lower split for your weekly routine rather than just building one area if you are not already. Sure, if you want bigger shoulders or more development in your legs, you will need to condition that area more, but that doesn't mean you should neglect other body parts.

Keep in mind where your weak spots are and train accordingly. If you experience pain in your elbows, make sure you pay extra attention to form in exercises such as the bench press or dips and think about investing in some elbow supports. There is no shame in wearing protective gear, and you don't need to worry about what other people will think. However, it's also important you seek medical help for joint pains or anything like that since you need to know where the pain is coming from. You don't want to continue training only to find out you have worsened a condition.

One of the great things about using the gym is there are infinite ways to activate your muscles. Invest the time into learning about your body and then work around those limitations.

Now let's look at how we can add even more intensity in the gym or at home with a clear strategy and approach to our workouts.

6

HIIT FOR 50-AND-ABOVE STRENGTH WARRIORS

Have you heard of HIIT? You most probably have. We touched on this lightly in a previous chapter, and this time around, we will dive deep and give you a better understanding of what it is and how to make the most of it.

HIIT CULTURE

For some reason, the HIIT system is gaining more popularity with the younger crowd. Maybe it's because the matured ladies and gentlemen of today are too busy to spend time learning all the new fitness trends, or perhaps it's because they prefer doing things the old way. In either case, they are missing out on the benefits of this training system. On the other hand, you could

144 | BRYANT WILLIS

already be well aware of this technique, in which case I am here to help sharpen your knowledge on the subject and give you a better understanding.

High-Intensity Interval Training (HIIT) is precisely what the name suggests. It consists of putting several workouts together in the form of a circuit acting at a fast pace. These can be bodyweight exercises or performed with weights; the aim is to do them in quick succession. The circuit is centered around time and efficiency rather than getting a certain number of reps in. Essentially a circuit consists of several exercises, while a set only contains one or two exercises. However, the main difference is the way it's performed.

Some of the most familiar concerns and questions I receive include:

- Does HIIT have any substantial benefits for me as an older athlete?
- How do I fit high-intensity interval training into my routine?
- HIIT looks intense and fast-paced. Is this safe for me to do?
- Why is everyone getting into HIIT?

I'll try my best to answer all of your concerns and queries.

Why You Should Consider HIIT

These are valid concerns, and I believe we should always question the legitimacy of new ways of training. Moreover, humans are creatures of habit; when we find something that works reasonably well, it's hard to branch out at the risk of wasting our energy. I'm sure many of you have been doing the same routine for quite some time now, and it has become second nature.

The question is, how effective is your strategy, and could you be missing out on potential gains?

This is where a lot of traditionalists start to get nervous. Yes, change is daunting if you feel comfortable and knowledgeable about what you're doing, although adaptation is essential if it can help you.

1. How do we know that our training gives us the best possible development for both strength and muscle growth?

Naturally, most people will think that if a session leaves you sore the next day, it's working. They equate muscle soreness to muscle damage and muscle damage to muscle growth.

But let's consider the example of marathon runners. They cause a lot of muscle damage in a single run, yet they don't have very muscular legs. Instead, most long-distance runners have very slender legs. According to the commonly held belief, these runners should have giant legs, shouldn't they?

There is mounting evidence to support the fact that not all muscle damage results in muscle growth. Surprisingly, it's found that muscle damage can result in muscle atrophy, AKA muscle loss. When we look to gain mass, we need to induce a certain kind of stress on the muscle, leading to growth later on. Simply working out longer, doing more reps with more weight is not the solution. Techniques and efficiency are far more superior.

BENEFITS OF HIIT

When we consider overall health, your metabolism plays a significant role in how well your body performs. HIIT helps improve your metabolic rate. It's is structured to kick start even the slowest metabolisms and keep you at an elevated rate for several hours after the workout. Meaning all processes in your body are actually working at a much higher rate; this includes protein synthesis, digestion, muscle growth, and even brain function.

Another major benefit is that HIIT allows you to shed the right kind of weight. When you're losing weight, it's not always fat. In most cases, you will lose a combination of fat and the precious muscle you have spent years training for. Through HIIT, you can optimize that weight loss process and prepare your body to offload the fat without sacrificing the good stuff.

As you may have noticed in half the exercises discussed so far, they are large compound movements requiring you to be strong in all areas to perform efficiently. A weakness in any one area can make the exercise far more challenging to execute. It would help if you had a healthy amount of flexibility, balance, and strength to perform these workouts. HIIT enables you to improve all these areas and develop a more functional physique that will pave the way for more potential gains.

Last but not least is the improvement in cardiovascular health that HIIT gives you. Rather than having to do mind-numbing hours of cardio on the treadmill, a solid HIIT workout is going to provide you with a much better cardio workout in a much shorter time. Whether you aim to lose weight or improve your endurance, you can undoubtedly get these cardio gains through HIIT.

But wait, I'm a strength athlete. I need fine-cut muscles, not stamina!

If you don't have the mortar, how do you expect to stack the bricks without collapsing? In other words, how are you hoping to get the kind of strength gains you want without a strong heart, healthy lungs, and a capable body? Without proper body conditioning, you are limiting the amount of training you can do. Eventually, this will limit the kind of progress you can make.

HIIT is more than just developing stamina; it is about muscle conditioning and generating explosive and functional power. Unless you are planning on going professional and making money from strength training, chances are you want to live better and add an extra ten years to your life, rather than just being able to bench all the plates at your local gym.

Simply getting around can be a bother for people in their '70s and even '60s. Putting in the effort today will allow you to enjoy the benefits of a happier life to the very end.

GETTING STARTED WITH HIIT

At its core, the concept of high-intensity interval training is straightforward and can be implemented in various ways. Many of the exercises used in HIIT are the same workouts as what you have previously learned.

We have covered the basic bodyweight exercises and free weight exercises in the previous book. We have gone through some advanced bodyweight activities in this installment, and they can all be fused into a solid HIIT workout. You could even throw in those lat pull-downs or any other machine-oriented movement that we discussed. However, speed is a crucial component for high-intensity interval training, so that is why I advise you to stick with bodyweight movements. You don't want to get caught out adjusting a cable machine while in the middle of your circuit. As long as the activity is a compound movement that recruits a lot of muscle fiber, I would consider it for HIIT. The only thing you don't want to be doing is minimal, concentrated exercises like bicep curls or calf raise; Although they are superb at building hypertrophy for a compact area, the rest of the body is left to sit idle.

Also, when it comes to creating more advanced HIIT circuits, you can do this by simply employing some of the high-intensity techniques that we discussed earlier.

More reps in each set, more sets in the same time frame, lower rest intervals, etc., all these are simple ways to take the intensity a notch higher on HIIT circuits. Moreover, you can incorporate different exercises. Rather than just relying on bodyweight workouts, you can bring in free weight exercises, so long as it doesn't require much preparation. It's like putting together a well-prepared meal; you can use any ingredient you like as long as you time everything perfectly.

Adding Some Spice To HIIT

To give you some extra oomph, here are a few effective exercises to get the blood pumping in your HIIT program. Not only are these highly intense exercises, but when you do them back-to-back with some high-intensity strategies, they can prove to be a killer.

Push Ups - but they aren't enough this time.

Push-Ups are central in any calisthenics program, military fitness test, and even cross-fit competition because they are a tested measure of strength. Moreover, you can add weights to these in the form of plates on your back, you can change the way your hands are placed on the floor, you can do clapping push-ups, and the list goes on. This is one of those exercises that you can do a hundred ways, and they will all be beneficial. I feel confident in saying I don't need to explain in detail how to perform this movement so let's skip over that part and talk about how we can make it exceedingly challenging. Combine push-up variations with your burpees, and now you get an exercise that reaches all the major muscles in your body while pushing your fitness levels to the limit - a necessary asset in your HIIT arsenal.

Something to keep in mind with the push-up; some people tend to go all the way down till their chest bumps the ground, this might look intense, but it takes all the tension off your muscles. This method is not good form, nor is it suitable for muscle stimulation.

I understand that some of you have arthritis in your wrists, and this can limit you from performing the standard push-up as it puts the wrist in a compromising position. But I have the solution, and it comes at a reasonable cost. I urge you to invest in some push-up handles, also known as push-up bars. For $10, you can acquire a pair of these and continue without experiencing pain in your wrists. If you are wondering, you place these little metal hoops on the floor and grip them at the top; this way, you don't have to hyperextend your wrist and potentially injure it. I promise that I don't have a partnership deal with any brands, but I swear by this equipment because it has personally helped one of my clients/friends regain the ability to perform push-ups. If you are proficient with push-ups and don't experience any pain, then take it to the next level with your feet up on a bench so that your body is on a decline. You can also use chains around your neck, wear a weighted vest or even hold bands around your shoulders and tuck them under your hand to provide additional resistance in the movement, although I don't think you will need it.

The three variations I suggest are as follows:

- Standard push-ups
- Wide push-ups
- Diamond push-ups

Cycle through these push-ups after every burpee until the time runs out, and you feel the effects of full-body activation.

Jumping Jacks - to the extreme

Some people also know these as star jumps. A familiar movement we all know too well. Unfortunately for someone like you, this basic movement isn't enough to get your blood pumping, so we are upgrading to Squat Jacks. This adaptation makes all the difference, so don't be surprised if your legs are quivering after a thorough session. I'll go through it step-by-step so you can effectively fuse these two exercises into a quad destroyer.

1. We begin this movement in the standard squat position with your knees bent, back straight, and pelvis sticking out.
2. From here, create tension in your body and explode up. Your feet should come together, and hands should swing over your body until they touch at the top.

3. In quick succession, you need to hop back to the squat position and lower yourself.

The entire movement should be swift, with the only exception when you lower down for a squat. This action should be controlled; otherwise, the exercise won't be effective, and you could potentially injure your knee caps.

This three-step action completes one rep of the squat jack. To increase resistance, you can easily add additional weight by wearing a weighted jacket. Another purpose would be to do a few of these before your main workout as a high-intensity warm-up.

Mountain Climbers - with some help from the obliques

When doing mountain climbers, it is crucial to keep in mind that this is a CORE exercise. It helps to maintain that mind-to-muscle connection and focus on the movement to maximize stress on your core rather than other areas of the body. Your legs and arms play a role in this movement but don't forget your objective.

As I mentioned earlier, we want to try and include as much muscle activation as we can when doing HIIT. So, to achieve greater activation of the midsection, we will use the Cross-Body Climber variation; this will bring your obliques into the picture and increase difficulty - here is how you do it.

1. Start at the top of a push-up position. Keep everything nice and straight from your shoulders to your hip and glutes to your ankles, paying extra attention to your lower back and hips. This exercise will focus on your core; keeping your hips too far up will limit the tension on your abs.
2. Bring one knee up and slightly touch your elbow. Squeeze with your core muscles and return that knee to the starting position. Every other body part should remain still except your leg and the rotation of your hips.
3. The aim is not to do this fast; you aren't running against the floor. The objective is to get the entire core to move your knee towards your chest. When you rotate, you don't want to place tension on your shoulders or lower back, just the abdominals and obliques.

This is a fantastic exercise that will help you build that core strength that you need for deadlifts, squats, and nearly everything else. The issue is, most people don't get the benefits of this exercise because they cheat and jump into the position. Adding rotation will minimize this but let me emphasize that the only thing moving should be your hips and your knees. Try to make this a priority.

Pull-Up

This is another potent exercise that is excellent for HIIT workouts. However, we have covered pull-ups extensively in a previous chapter, so further information is redundant.

Nevertheless, I highly recommend getting a portable pull-up bar that you can set up at home, so you don't have to rely on a gym. It's an inexpensive piece of equipment that has tremendous value.

Burpee Box Jumps

A lower body killer. If you have absolutely no time and want to do something that will get the blood flowing, get the muscles burning, and do everything else you could want from a workout, this one exercise is the answer. This combination of two critical leg exercises will give your muscle a workout to remember.

1. Start in a standing position with your arms at your sides and your feet roughly shoulder-width apart.
2. Squat down to your hands while

simultaneously kicking your legs out behind you as if you are jumping into a push-up stance.

3. From this position, perform a standard push-up.

4. On your way back up, bring both feet back towards your chest.

5. As you are bringing your legs back in, shift the weight from your hands to your feet so you can explode upwards.

6. From this position, explode vertically off your feet and onto the platform. Then, instead of jumping off the platform and potentially damaging your knees, lower your body with a squat and then hop off the platform. This will lessen the impact on your body.

It might sound like a lot to do, but when you understand the flow of this movement, it's very natural, very smooth, but highly challenging. Especially if you are wearing a training vest or focusing on speed, it's intense on the muscles and the cardiovascular system. It is a complete workout that you can do wherever you are, whenever you have a few minutes.

Side Plank Thread The Needle

For the side plank Thread The Needle (TTN), you want to make sure you have some cushioning for your elbow as all your weight will be on one side.

1. Start by laying on the ground at your side. Have your feet stacked one on top of the other and hold yourself up with your forearm flat to the ground just like if you were laying in bed on your side watching TV.
2. Now, lift your hip off the floor with your core - maintain a good posture, keeping everything straight down to your feet. Make sure your elbow is directly underneath your shoulder.
3. Raise your other arm straight into the air and extend it out as high as you can reach while keeping everything tight.
4. Imagine that you are holding a thread in your fingers on the hand that is extended. The needle hole you need to thread this through is the space underneath your torso. You want to bring your arm down and poke it through this triangular gap between your other arm.
5. The key is to make sure you don't sink into your shoulder, as this will cause your hips to lower and break posture.

Keeping your elbow and hips high is the essence of this movement, and if done right, this exercise will be fantastic for building stability and rotational ability.

PUTTING HIIT INTO ACTION

HIIT is one of those things that you can easily overdo. Since the workouts are so short, people usually overdo the training because they feel they haven't fully exerted enough energy.

Work And Rest

As a general rule of thumb, you should remember that a longer work session is better for building endurance, while shorter/more intense work sessions are more effective for building strength. So if you were training for a marathon, you would be doing a HIIT circuit that required you to work for 60 seconds and rest for 30, while if you were training for strength, you would work for 30 seconds and rest for 60.

It's also important to understand that not all forms of rest are the same. For instance, are you just sitting down on a bench after an exercise and sipping some ice water, or are you doing a slow walk on the treadmill? Having some form of movement during rest can assist in the removal of lactic acid from the muscle and help you recover faster.

Intensity

It would be best if you also considered the intensity with which you will be working out. Exerting too little energy will not give you the best result from HIIT, and going too hard may result in total fatigue before the session is complete. If you are going too hard or too heavy in the session, you won't maintain solid form, which will result in a higher risk of injury. The solution is to find that sweet spot where you are giving every-thing you have at such a pace that you can sustain it for the entirety of the session while having enough strength to perform everything correctly. Ideally, a good HIIT session should be very challenging, not exhausting to the point that you can't walk around.

The best way to gauge the sweet spot of intensity is to have a specific heart rate that you want to achieve and then maintain throughout the session. To achieve this, first, we need to know your maximum heart rate to determine your limit. Here is the formula: 220 - your age = (MHR) your maximum heart rate. We can use a heart rate monitor to measure how hard you should be pushing yourself now that we know your MHR.

- Aim between 60 to 70 percent of your MHR in the first 5 minutes of the workout.
- Then progress to 80 to 90 percent, as long as you can sustain it between 30 seconds to a couple of minutes, depending on your fitness levels.
- At this point, your body will need to recover, so

slow down and aim to hit between 40 and 50 percent of your MHR for roughly 3 minutes before repeating this cycle.

Volume

Then there is also the question of volume. How much work should you be doing per session? Again, this is something that only you are going to understand when you start a HIIT protocol. Don't get discouraged if you can't complete the first workout; it's your body telling you to reduce the overall volume next time and possibly lower the resistance. I always advise people to start small and build their way up. As you feel more confident in your ability to continue, you can always add an extra exercise or another lap of the circuit.

HIIT IN PRACTICE

Here is a short and speedy HIIT workout session that I will share with you to give you an idea of what HIIT looks like in action.

This whole workout should only take about 15 minutes, including rest. That's all it takes to burn a ton of calories and kick start your metabolism. We will use some of the exercises we discussed, so you have the chance to learn them.

1. Squat Jacks

Work – 20 sec, rest – 30 sec

Using the technique you've learned, simply blast your heels from the deep squat position to launch yourself into the air. Land gently on your feet and move straight into the next squat.

2. Burpee Box Jump

Work – 20 sec, Rest – 10 sec

Have the platform ready to go before starting this workout, so you are not wasting any time.

3. Cross-Body Climber

Work – 20 sec, Rest – 10 sec

Get in position and alternate knees with every rep, keeping your core nice and tight.

Repeat this 3-exercise circuit 8 times, and that's it. Your rest time in-between circuit is up to you but try not to take longer than one and a half minutes. Also, keep your eyes on your heart monitor to evaluate the intensity, as we discussed earlier.

PROPER USAGE OF HIIT

As the name suggests, HIIT is all about intensity, explosiveness, and turbo-charged energy. Even though this is fantastic for cardio and strength, it needs to be used with care and caution. Since it is very explosive, there is a high chance of injury if you don't have the proper form dialed in your brain. Moreover, when you are doing things at close to maximum capacity, you exert a lot more stress and pressure on your body, so an injury can be pretty serious during these exercises. I would highly suggest ensuring you are in a suitable physical and mental condition before performing a HIIT session.

Sometimes if you don't feel in top shape, maybe you haven't slept well, or the last couple of days at work have been exhausting. There is nothing wrong with skipping a HIIT session and just doing regular, low-intensity cardio.

I would also like to point out that HIIT supplements your basic strength training; it's not a replacement. Just because you are doing HIIT doesn't mean you can skip everything else.

This brings us to one of the most critical points: incorporating HIIT into your workout regime effectively. First off, you don't want to pair HIIT sessions on the same days as your strength training day. They are both high-energy workouts, and doing one will not leave you with enough energy for the other. Do HIIT on a day when you have no other plans for exercise, and ideally in-between rest days.

Secondly, HIIT is not a regular training system. For the best results, you should be using this one or twice a week, no more. Especially if you are doing other strength training work, you don't need more than 2 HIIT sessions in a week, nor can your body afford it. Also, keep each HIIT session at least 48 hours apart. The EPOC effect can last anywhere from 24 hours to 48 hours after a HIIT session. You want EPOC to have completely worn off before you do any more.

In my own experience and through vigorous HIIT research, doing too much of it will be catabolic. The extreme energy requirements will naturally impact your muscle mass. Even though you will be losing weight, much of that weight will be muscle.

When your body is in an energy-hungry state, it needs fuel. Even though you are eating well, both foods in your belly and the fat around your body slowly release energy stores. After HIIT, your body needs fuel quickly, and the fastest energy store is through the muscle. Balancing out your weekly routine will make sure your body is not doing itself harm.

Where do I fit HIIT into my week?

If you are pondering the idea of adding HIIT into your weekly routine, then I would suggest doing regular workout routines the majority of the week and diving into HIIT once or twice. For example, you could work your upper body on Monday then rest the following day before doing HIIT on Wednesday. Then switch to your lower body routine on Friday after a day of rest.

TOP TIPS

The most important thing is proper execution and proper form during these exercises. Especially when you are going through a HIIT circuit, you will notice that lactic acid builds up much faster, you get out of breath much quicker, and your muscles get depleted of energy at a higher rate. All these things contribute significantly to poor form and half-hearted movements.

When you lose form, you begin losing potential gains. There is no point in doing these exercises, or any activities for that matter, with poor form. If you aren't getting the full range of motion, if you aren't placing the required stress on your muscles, then you aren't training.

As a wise man once said

'Just because you are doing a lot more doesn't mean you are getting a lot more done. Don't confuse movement with progress.'

— **DENZEL WASHINGTON**

Training your body is just as much a mental workout as it is a physical one. You don't want to be going through the motions without thought; you want to be engaged in the activity, and consciously taking the steps that you trust will give you a better body.

THE FINAL COUNTDOWN

What started as some basic exercises in 'The Seven Keys To Strength Training For Men Over 50' grew into more advanced practices in this book's earlier portion. Later on, we looked at taking the intensity up a notch by adding some high-intensity systems. We added some diversity by throwing in some weight training and understanding how to have fun while doing business in the gym.

This chapter looks at how you can take all those exercises and systems and compress them into an even more intense HIIT protocol to get even better results. I want to add that to get the most out of HIIT; you need to take it slow and steady. I realize that this will be a learning curve for most people who have been using traditional training systems for most of their lives, so take the time to understand what you are doing.

It's also essential not to forget the importance of rest, nutrition, and sufficient recovery. More literature suggests that even though HIIT facilitates better recovery due to several factors, training more than four times a week with a high-intensity training system leads to a loss of muscle mass and hinders overall performance.

On the contrary, short, explosive workouts of approximately 20-30 minutes each done three times a week yield the best results. So have fun with these systems but remember that they serve a very functional purpose, and to get the most out of them, you need to be honest with yourself.

With your rest, recovery, and exercises out of the way, let's look at how you can set yourself up for success and design a fit lifestyle that you will be happy to maintain for the rest of your life.

7

STAYING ON TRACK; STAYING MOTIVATED

WHY STOP?

I specialize in training middle-aged to aged ladies and gentlemen, I work with clients over the age of 40, but I'm very familiar with younger people and how they train. I can tell you from experience that many of the older gents that I coach are in much better physical condition than some of the younger guys I see in the gym.

Problems such as obesity, high blood pressure, heart disease, and even mobility problems are just as prevalent in younger people.

These things generally affect people later in life, but you would be surprised to see how many young people are dealing with these issues today.

There are multiple reasons for this, and the two that stand out the most are a poor diet and a sedentary lifestyle.

Humans were not designed to sit behind a desk for 9 hours a day and look at a screen. So, for those of you who do your best to maintain good health, you deserve a pat on the back.

You should be very proud of how much effort you put into your physical health, and a comforting thought is knowing you are already doing better than the average person.

Use this as fuel and be freed, knowing that the effects of age will always be inadequate compared to hard work. If you feel low or doubt your ability to be better, know that you are among a small, elite group of people, people who are willing to walk the path of self-improvement. So, do not worry if the road is hard; if it weren't, everyone would be perfect. To think that no one on this earth is perfect should give you clarity and confidence that every small step forward is a testament to your character.

If things are going well for you, congratulations, but be prepared for those physical and mental slumps that we all encounter. It may be a problem with your day job, it might be an injury, or it could be a sudden change in your life. Whenever the world throws you off track, remember, you can handle it. The superpower of being middle-aged to older is that you have been through it all and seen it all. Getting this far in life has hardened you into an unbreakable beast, and I sincerely envy that.

COMMON CHALLENGES

Whether you are a dad looking to get in shape for your kid's wedding, a woman returning to the gym after decades of restless work, or a person getting into the gym for the first time, there are a few common problems we all face. I want to share my thoughts, so they might help you get over these bumps in the road.

Plateaus

Simply put, this is a phase most of us will experience at some point along the way. You have been training hard and eating right, but your body stops giving you the response you're looking for. Don't let this get to you; we all face it, and there are multiple ways around it that I will discuss later on.

Injuries

Another monotonous problem we all face. While dealing with the injury is a challenge in itself, it can be tough to get the engines going after weeks or possibly months of sitting idle. The longer you are out, the harder it will be, but it's not impossible. Unfortunately, your muscles will be considerably weaker because we lose muscle strength rapidly. However, all is not lost; thankfully, our muscles do not degenerate as quickly as our strength, so start with lower resistance, and soon your strength will catch up.

Boredom

Even professional athletes will tell you they don't always enjoy working out. This is why it's good to set small, achievable goals along the way, so our brain receives a nice dose of dopamine every time we pass one - this could be as small as increasing your bench-press by 5 pounds.

Distractions

Life is constantly throwing a series of figurative busses at your door. Distractions are usually the cause of laziness. We let our focus drift onto indulging in useless pleasures like watching the entire Lord Of The Rings franchise in one sitting. We are creatures of habit, so it's imperative to stay on your schedule and get your workout in when it's due. Putting it off till later often means you miss that day. That day quickly becomes a week, then a month, and when you look in the mirror, you are back where you started.

SOLUTIONS TO COMMON CHALLENGES

When I see people who have lost interest, it's because they have hit a plateau in many cases. This leads to boredom, which leads to them eventually falling off track.

When they started, they saw gains, which then motivated them to carry on.

However, these things soon start to slow down till; eventually, there comes the point where it becomes a lot harder to make progress, and diet has to be considered.

This is a training plateau and something that we have to overcome strategically.

If you are currently facing this problem, this will not be the first time, nor will it be the last. These are going to happen many times, and it is something that even elite-level athletes struggle with. So please don't give up and read on to find my top tips for overcoming this problem.

There are a few reasons why this may be happening to you.

You may be overtraining

Believe it or not, sometimes pushing your body too hard can limit development. Especially if you lack other vital areas such as rest and diet, your body can quickly sink into a fatigued state of being. While you might feel full of energy, your body doesn't have the fuel to induce more growth.

Consider taking a few days off, increasing your food intake and amount of sleep, or cutting down on training to give your body a chance to recover.

You may not be training enough

Just like the concept of Ying and Yang, you must try to find the right balance. Beginner gains can be misleading. When you first start after a long break, you will see incredible gains; this can mislead you into training lighter, slacking off on a diet, and cutting corners in the fitness plan. If this sounds like you, I advise you to take greater action into your fitness journey, as a half-hearted attempt isn't going to cut it anymore.

You may be overeating

Some people actually gain weight when they start training because they feel like they need to eat more since they are working out. They aren't consciously going for seconds and thirds, but since their body is demanding more energy they are consuming more than is necessary. This is especially true in the case of people who are already supposed to be in a calorie deficit.

You may not be eating enough

Some people experience an expanded appetite when they go all-in. They aren't consciously greedy, but since their bodies demand more energy, they consume more without thinking about it. Although it is essential to know your daily food intake and plan accordingly, putting the right foods in your body is of greater importance. By eating the right stuff like slow-release carbs, your body will use the energy more effectively. If you want to expand your knowledge on proper diet, I recommend downloading my free One Day Weight Loss Meal Plan. You can download it by following the instructions at the very beginning of this book.

You may be eating the wrong things

In a hurry to see rapid fat loss, or because of a hectic schedule, you might not be eating enough. It's easy to underestimate the value of good food. Protein shakes and supplements will not replace real food, and you need to give your body enough building blocks to help it create a masterpiece. If you are short of time or suffer from a small appetite, consider adding small, healthy snacks to your day in between your three main meals. Snacking won't do you any harm so long as you eat the right food.

You're not giving your body enough time to rest and recuperate

This is especially true in the case of people using HIIT extensively. It would be best if you gave your body enough time to recover and grow back before you can start breaking it down again. This is where a bit of foresight and long-term thinking will be beneficial; sometimes, it is better to take a day off at the expense of losing momentum than to burn out and lose a month of training.

You are under stress from other aspects of your life – job, family, money, etc

A common problem. We aren't professional athletes who have nothing else to do but spend hours in the gym. We all have countless other things going on in life. Stress and anxiety can considerably impact our bodies and the kind of progress we can make in the gym. Unfortunately, there is no easy way around this problem because you will always have something on your plate. That said, I believe the best way is to organize your week through compromise. Make compromise your best friend. If you agree to meet your friend on a day you are supposed to work out, decide to shorten your time together and do a brief workout at the gym after. There are only so many hours in the day, so adapting is the only way to remain satisfied.

Losing motivation

If you find it hard to get out of bed to go for your morning run, if you don't feel like getting up and creating a healthy meal, if you feel like staying at home on your day off and doing nothing, chances are you're just like everyone else.

You have to realize that it's completely fine to be in that state of mind, but actions speak louder than words, and it isn't acceptable to live in that mindset. Even professional athletes will tell you there are days when they don't want to do it, but they do it anyway.

It's not reasonable to expect yourself to be motivated every day, but if you can break the default setting in your head, that is how the greats are made, and that's how you separate from your past self.

Why did you get into strength training? Look back at your goals and look forward to your ambitions.

The Cookie Jar

This is a great mental exercise that can help you on so many levels in such a powerful way. There are two ways to do it.

Positive

When you are feeling low, I want you to think of your dreams, ambitions, desires, and all those things that fill your head with joy. If you could write these things down on a piece of paper, this will help you focus and give you a list that you can refer to later. And don't worry, this isn't some voodoo, star reeding bs okay. Scientific studies have shown that writing something down can help you remember it better, and that's all I want you to do.

When you are pushing through those last few reps, think of giving up, when you don't want to get out of bed, and all those breaking points you will encounter, please think of all those dreams. Think of all those things that could help you and your family in the future. Even though working out might not directly correlate, know that triumphing with your fitness will lead to more wins in your life, as you have acquired the drive to put in the work.

Every rep is another move towards making those thoughts a reality.

Negative

Similarly, you could compile a list of things you have overcome or something you dislike about the past. These are all the negative people in your life, the unfortunate events, and all kinds of pain you have felt.

When life gets tough, think of all those people who said you couldn't do it, think of those times when the world seemed like it was over, think of that negativity, and whack on some music as you fight back through shire will power. Each rep is an F you to negative people. Each workout is a big step forward and an opportunity to laugh at that negativity and prove that you can do better. If you can learn to channel your emotions into motivation, there is no limit to what you can accomplish.

STAY ON TOP OF YOUR MIND

I want to remind you that your perspective has a massive impact on your life. It can be your demise or your uprising, but one of the greatest gifts bestowed upon humans is the ability to change our minds. It is the only thing we have control over, so I urge you to use it.

It would help if you remembered that the path of least resistance is the path of no progress. To make changes in your life, you need to accept that there will be many times when you are uncomfortable.

However, learning to be comfortable in uncomfortable situations is a superpower that you can acquire.

Before we conclude this book, I wanted to say a few words. First of all, how proud I am that you could remain focused on your goal right up until the very last word. It might not seem like a big deal right now, and you may have blitzed through this book in a mere day but let me remind you how important this is.

By finishing this book, you have taken the correct steps in becoming a better you. A stronger you, both physically and mentally, and I genuinely hope you enjoyed the ride.

If you found enjoyment reading this book or learned anything helpful along the way, I ask only one thing. Let me know your appreciation by writing a short review on amazon. Most people might not realize, but reviews are the lifeline of all books on Amazon; they are the difference between a happy ending and a failed dream. I understand people are busy, but it would be greatly appreciated if you could find the time to show your appreciation. Here's how you do it...

Head over to Amazon.com or Amazon.co.uk, depending on where you are located.

Then look over in the top right where it says "returns and orders" on desktop, or if you are using mobile, then hit the little person icon in the top right of your screen and then hit "track and manage your orders."

From there, it's really easy; on desktop, it should say "write a product review," and for mobile, you need to tap on the book, and it should come up with the same thing.

Thanks again, and now for some final words.

CONCLUSION

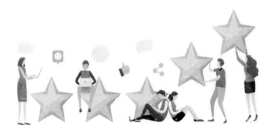

I believe we have the ability to change our quality of life.

For most people, it's about changing your mindset, a shift in perspective on how you see yourself.

You can tell better than I can just how different your body is from 20 years ago. You have a first-hand understanding of what time can do to your body, but the astonishing part is you can reverse these effects with the right knowledge.

I'm not saying you can go back to your 18-year-old body, but I am saying that things you thought were no longer possible are utterly possible if you are willing to put in the work. I'm sure by now you are well aware of this, although I like to bring it up in hopes of reinvigorating your passion for exercise.

You can still hike, you can still enjoy food, you can still move the iron in the gym and enjoy life to the fullest. The only thing that has changed over the years is your wisdom and knowledge.

Over the course of this book, I hope I have successfully shown you that getting your ideal body and maintaining it doesn't require a million-dollar home gym investment or a ten thousand dollar trainer. It requires a will to change and guidance to help you implement daily practices that inch you closer to a better life.

Understand that working out is not enough. Your body is an ecosystem, it has a variety of requirements, and when it comes to health, you have to give it the fuel that it needs, the time it wants, and the stimulation it requires.

You will notice the wonders a healthy diet can do for your body, not only for your fitness but for other areas like mood and quality of life.

Note that change is necessary, but drastic change is a form of chaos, so there is no need to put this book down and go for an hour-long run. Instead, it would be best if you were looking to take gradual steps that chip away at the issues you face.

Things like better sleeping habits are going to help you in many areas outside of the gym. I understand that we all have different schedules and different routines, but sleep, exercise, and food are the basics that no one should avoid under any circumstance.

This ecosystem that we call our body is always running, and if you want to make your existence better, it's best to start with your internal environment.

Throughout this book, we have covered many ways to start making changes today, in fact, right now. You can get exceptional results with bodyweight exercises, and trust me, that is all that's required for many people. If you've ever had a chance to meet a marine, a navy seal, or anyone in the Special Forces, I can assure you that they rely on calisthenics (bodyweight exercises) more than weight training. As a marine, physical conditioning is just as vital as mental conditioning; it's how they can build the resilience to get through the hard times.

This is not to discount the fact that working out in the gym is also highly beneficial.

If you are already training and are looking to take things to the next level, then pay attention to what we have discussed regarding intensity. Again, these things can get complicated, and it can be risky when working with heavy weights, so having some assistance always helps.

Adding intensity will undoubtedly help you break through any plateaus you have, whether mental or physical. If training is starting to get tedious and you can't find it in yourself to get back to the gym, look into HIIT; maybe this will revive your excitement for training. Not only is it an extraordinarily fast-paced and mentally stimulating workout, but it's also a holistic approach to physical fitness. It's going to put you through your paces for both strength and cardio if you use it right.

Lastly, let me rephrase something you already know, there will be rainy days. Proper planning, proper education of movements, and understanding your body will help minimize the possibility of injury. Still, there will be rainy days, whether a training injury, a professional hurdle or a problem in your personal life. It's okay to take some time off if it's justified, but eventually, try to ease back into your life's routine because that is the only thing that will make you happier. Having a fit body gives you a strong mind, and those two elements combined won't make problems easier, but it will increase the chances of you getting back up and brushing it off.

I have seen so many people fighting depression, anxiety, stress, and all sorts of other problems, and getting in better shape has completely changed their perspective. It has transformed how they see themselves, which has made all the difference.

Take the knowledge from this book and apply it to your life today to live a more stimulating, healthier, and happier life.

I'd love to hear from you, but unfortunately, we may never meet. I want you to go out there today, cook yourself a healthy dinner, go out for a short walk, get back in the gym and hit those weights, and then come back and drop a review on this book, explaining how it has helped you, along with a message about what you have done to be better.

Time to warm up.

REFERENCES

Guerin, G. (2015, April 20). Lifting at any age has rewards, but after 50 it can change your life. Retrieved November 11, 2021, from nj website: https://www.nj.com/healthfit/fitness/2015/04/post_49.html

(2017, November 23). Why you should see your doctor before starting an exercise program. Retrieved November 11, 2021, from Drdavidgeier.com website: https://www.drdavidgeier.com/see-your-doctor/

DeNoon, D. J. (2007, July 16). Weight training for heart disease. Retrieved November 11, 2021, from WebMD website: https://www.webmd.com/heart-disease/news/20070716/weight-training-for-heart-disease

Basaraba, S. (n.d.). Common age-related diseases and conditions. Retrieved November 11, 2021, from Verywellhealth.com website: https://www.verywellhealth. com/age-related-diseases-2223996

5 weight training tips for people with arthritis. (2021, February 3). Retrieved November 11, 2021, from Harvard.edu website: https://www.health.harvard.edu/ staying-healthy/5-weight-training-tips-for-people-with-arthritis

Deer, R. R., & Volpi, E. (2015). Protein intake and muscle function in older adults. *Current Opinion in Clinical Nutrition and Metabolic Care, 18*(3), 248–253.

Simmonds, K. (2021, July 24). Nutrition for seniors: What to know. Retrieved November 11, 2021, from Cynicalsenior.com website: https://cynicalsenior.com/ nutrition-for-seniors-what-to-know/

Whey protein shakes may help build muscle mass in seniors. (2017, July 25). Retrieved November 11, 2021, from Healthline Media website: https://www. healthline.com/health-news/whey-protein-shakes-may-help-build-muscle-mass-in-seniors

Preserve your muscle mass. (2016, February 19). Retrieved November 11, 2021, from Harvard.edu website: https://www.health.harvard.edu/staying-healthy/preserve-your-muscle-mass

TheRobertsonTrainingSystems/timeline. (2021, September 24). The science of muscle recovery: How long should you rest between workouts? Retrieved November 11, 2021, from Bodybuilding.com website: https://www.bodybuilding.com/content/the-science-of-muscle-recovery-how-long-should-you-rest-between-workouts.html

Waehner, P. (n.d.). Progressive Resistance for Strength Training. Retrieved November 11, 2021, from Very-wellfit.com website: https://www.verywellfit.com/progressive-resistance-1229835

Kuslikis, T. (2021, August 21). Top 100 hardest body-weight exercises of all time (updated 2021). Retrieved November 11, 2021, from Ashotofadrenaline.net website: https://ashotofadrenaline.net/hardest-bodyweight-exercises/

Theunissen, S. (2020, May 1). Bodyweight workout: The ultimate home workout solution. Retrieved November 11, 2021, from Workoutplan.org website: https://workoutplan.org/bodyweight-workout/

Muscle diagrams of major muscles exercised in weight training. (2009, November 24). Retrieved November 11, 2021, from Motleyhealth.com website: https://www.motleyhealth.com/muscle-diagrams-of-major-muscles-exercised-in-weight-training

Rider, S. (2016, May 23). The bodyweight workout that builds big muscles. Retrieved November 11, 2021, from Coach website: https://www.coachmag.co.uk/fitness/workouts/bodyweight-workouts

(N.d.). Retrieved November 11, 2021, from Howtobeast.com website: https://www.howtobeast.com/3-reasons-full-body-routines-are-superior-to-split-routines/

Bornstein, A. (2021, May 17). How to overcome lost motivation. Retrieved November 11, 2021, from Bornfitness.com website: https://www.bornfitness.com/lost-motivation/

High-intensity interval training (HIIT): What it is, how to do it. (n.d.). Retrieved November 11, 2021, from Webmd.com website: https://www.webmd.com/fitness-exercise/a-z/high-intensity-interval-training-hiit

M&S Writers. (2008, May 8). 15 reasons why you're NOT building muscle! Retrieved November 11, 2021, from Muscleandstrength.com website: https://www.muscleandstrength.com/articles/why-youre-not-building-muscle.html

Warnock, M. (2020, March 15). HIIT workout for men over 50. Retrieved November 11, 2021, from Rocking50.com website: https://rocking50.com/hiit-workout-for-men-over-50/

(N.d.). Retrieved November 11, 2021, from Better-after50.com website: https://betterafter50.com/getting-fit-over-50-how-do-i-get-motivated/

Made in United States
North Haven, CT
28 January 2025

65014373R00117